# DATE DUE

| | | | |
|---|---|---|---|
| NO 17 '98 | DC 13 '04 | | |
| | JE 6 05 | | |
| DE 2 '98 | JE 4 06 | | |
| | AP 2 8 08 | | |
| DE 15 '99 | | | |
| AP 29 '99 | | | |
| DC 13 '99 | | | |
| NO 27 00 | | | |
| NY 25 00 | | | |
| DE 19 01 | | | |
| NY 15 02 | | | |
| JE 10 02 | | | |
| DE 2 02 | | | |
| JE 4 '03 | | | |
| DE 9 03 | | | |
| AP 17 04 | | | |

# Latina Adolescent Childbearing in East Los Angeles

R

# LATINA ADOLESCENT CHILDBEARING IN EAST LOS ANGELES

Pamela I. Erickson

 University of Texas Press, Austin

Requests for permission to reproduce material from this
work should be sent to Permissions, University of Texas
Press, P.O. Box 7819, Austin, TX 78713-7819.

∞The paper used in this publication meets the minimum
requirements of American National Standard for Information Sciences—Permanence of Paper for Printed
Library Materials, ANSI Z39.48-1984.

Library of Congress Cataloging-in-Publication Data
Erickson, Pamela I. (Pamela Irene), 1951 –
   Latina adolescent childbearing in East Los Angeles / Pamela I.
Erickson.
       p.   cm.
   Includes bibliographical references and index.
   ISBN 0-292-72093-9 (cloth : alk. paper).—ISBN 0-292-72094-7
(pbk. : alk. paper)
   1. Hispanic American teenage mothers—California—East Los
Angeles—Social conditions.   2. Hispanic American teenage
mothers—California—East Los Angeles—Family relationships.
3. Hispanic American men—California—East Los Angeles—Atti-
tudes.   4. Teenage pregnancy—California—East Los Angeles—
Prevention.   I. Title.
HQ759.4.E78   1998
306.874'3—dc21                                          97-30037

*To my grandmother Irene Sorensen Bemke;
my parents, Robert and Anna Erickson,
and my stepmother, Gladys Schaper; and
especially to my aunt Phyllis Nix Sorensen.*

# Contents

List of Figures      viii

List of Tables      ix

Preface      xi

Acknowledgments      xiii

Chapter 1. Introduction      1

Chapter 2. Culture, Norms, and Adolescent Childbearing      9

Chapter 3. The East Los Angeles Repeat-Pregnancy Prevention Project      35

Chapter 4. Los Angeles, the Hospital, and the Research Team      47

Chapter 5. The Latina Teen Mothers      62

Chapter 6. Prenatal Care and Birth Outcome      99

Chapter 7. Prevention of Repeat Pregnancy      114

Chapter 8. Contraceptive Use: The Intervening Variable      129

Chapter 9. Implications for America's War on Teenage Pregnancy      149

Postscript      165

Appendix A. Data-Collection Forms and Variables      167

Appendix B. Methods and Variable Definition for Quantitative Data      169

Notes      173

Bibliography      179

Index      191

# List of Figures

Figure 5.1. Two-Dimensional Multidimensional Scaling Plot of
Teens' Free Sort of Women's Roles                                    89

Figure 5.2. Two-Dimensional Multidimensional Scaling Plot of
Teens' Free Sort of Life Events                                      93

Figure 5.3. Schematic Contrast of the Ideal and Actual Life
Events for Teens                                                     95

Figure 8.1. Two-Dimensional Multidimensional Scaling Plots
of Providers' and Teens' Free Sort of Contraceptive
Methods                                                             139

Figure 8.2. Three-Dimensional Multidimensional Scaling Plot of
Teens' Free Sort of Contraceptive Methods                           140

# List of Tables

Table 2.1.  Median Age at Transition Events for American Women in 1988 — 16

Table 3.1.  Summary of Intervention Schedule for the 1989–1991 Hewlett Project — 41

Table 3.2.  Hewlett Project Recruitment, 1989–1991 — 41

Table 3.3.  Data-Collection Methods and Procedures, Hewlett Project, 1989–1991 — 42

Table 5.1.  Characteristics of Latina Teen Mothers 17 Years of Age and Under at LAC-USC Women's and Children's Hospital — 64

Table 5.2.  Country of Birth, Language, and Years in United States for Hewlett Project Participants — 65

Table 5.3.  Age, Pregnancy History, and Pregnancy Planning — 68

Table 5.4.  Education — 70

Table 5.5.  Relationship to Baby's Father — 78

Table 5.6.  Economic Support Expected from the Baby's Father — 82

Table 5.7.  Family Living in United States — 85

Table 5.8.  Perceived Social Support and Score — 85

Table 5.9.  Percentage of Group with Risk Factors at Entry into Teen Project — 87

Table 5.10. Percentage of Teens with Selected Plans and Goals for the Future — 88

Table 5.11. Mean Ranking of Roles — 91

Table 5.12. Life Events and Staging of Normative Order for American Script and for Latina Women — 93

Table 5.13. Ideal and Actual Order of Life Events for Teens
and Providers                                              94
Table 6.1.  Adequacy of Prenatal Care (Percentage)         101
Table 6.2.  Los Angeles County Health Facilities           103
Table 6.3.  Source of Prenatal Care (Percentage)           104
Table 6.4.  Regression Coefficients of Predictor Variables on
Birth Weight                                               107
Table 7.1.  Program Retention for Postpartum Teen Mothers   116
Table 7.2.  Contraception and Reproductive Plans           116
Table 7.3.  Mothers Returning for Postpartum Appointment   119
Table 7.4.  Retention in Teen Program                      122
Table 7.5.  Loss to Follow-up in the Two-Year Sample       122
Table 7.6.  Repeat Pregnancy within One and Two Years      127
Table 8.1.  Contraceptive Methods Used over Time           131
Table 8.2.  Percentage with Repeat Pregnancy by Contraceptive
Method Reported at Twelve-Month Follow-up                  132
Table 8.3.  English and Spanish Names of the Contraceptive
Methods Used in Pile Sorts and Ranking Exercises           138
Table 8.4.  Mean Rank Order of Use for Sixteen Methods
of Contraception                                           142

# Preface

A book is always a work in progress even though the study it is based on represents only a slice of time, in this case from 1989 to 1991. In the years between project implementation and publication of this book, many things have occurred to make information that was current during the study period dated by the time of publication. In particular, there have been massive changes in the Los Angeles County–University of Southern California health care system and in the attitudes and policies toward undocumented immigrants in California. I have noted the most important changes in the clinical setting in the text.

Since the project staff are so important to the success of an intervention like the one described in this book, I have taken care to describe the key staff members in Chapter 4 and to update important events in their lives in the Postscript.

# Acknowledgments

As is always true, this book would not have been possible without the support of many different individuals and institutions.

First, I would like to acknowledge the institutions that funded the different phases of the Teen Project: The William and Flora Hewlett Foundation, The Joseph Drown Foundation, The Los Angeles Women's Foundation, The California Community Foundation, and the Los Angeles Regional Family Planning Council, Inc. I would also like to acknowledge the University of Connecticut Research Foundation, which funded the 1992 study, and the National Institute of Child Health and Human Development, which funds my current research (R29HD32351), an extension of the qualitative work I began in these previous projects. I must also thank the Alan Guttmacher Institute and *Medical Anthropology* for allowing me to use portions of previously published works.

Second, I would like to acknowledge the clinical and administrative staff of the LAC-USC Family Planning Clinic for their constant support of the Teen Project and their willingness to go the extra mile for teen clients. I especially want to acknowledge all of the Teen Outreach Workers (TOWs), past and present; the student workers and volunteers; and the UCLA Public Health students, without whom neither the intervention project nor this book would have been possible. In the clinical setting, the burden of a research project can be overwhelming. Yet the extra paperwork, the necessity of learning about computers, and the extra time spent with me were all borne graciously by the staff. Their dedication to their young clients was a source of inspiration and a reminder that health care need not be devoid of humanity.

Many individuals provided intellectual and personal support both during the implementation of the Teen Project and the writing of this volume. Some are friends, some teachers, some colleagues, and some are all three. I particularly want to thank Margie Arviso, Stephen Beckerman, Gerald S. Bernstein, América Casillas, Lorinda Castañeda, Ana Díaz, Merrill Eisenberg,

W. Penn Handwerker, Pat Jamieson, Celia P. Kaplan, Siri L. Kjos, Alicia Mancillas, Ann McElroy, Laura Menoher, Nancy Moss, Carmen Muñoz, Goleth Orozco, Blanca Ovalle, Dora Luz Pérez, Luz Molina Pérez, Jorge Reyes, Eva Rodríguez, Susan C. M. Scrimshaw, William F. Stein, Patricia K. Townsend, and Shirley Wright. Special thanks go to my husband and son, William and Jacob Murrow, who were unfailing in their support.

I have a special intellectual debt to Kristin Luker, Constance Nathanson, and Laurie Zabin, whose careful work on adolescent sexuality, pregnancy, and childbearing have shaped my thinking over the years.

Finally, grateful thanks go to the young mothers who participated in the Teen Project. I only hope that this work will provide a better understanding of their lives and help shape a kinder, more relevant social policy regarding teenage motherhood.

# Latina Adolescent Childbearing in East Los Angeles

## CHAPTER ONE

# Introduction

This book is about teenage pregnancy among Latina adolescents in East Los Angeles, or as we call it, East L.A.[1] It focuses on teenage pregnancy and motherhood among economically disadvantaged Latinas aged 17 and under. The young mothers discussed herein and listed below were participants in a series of intervention efforts to prevent repeat pregnancy at the Family Planning Clinic at the Los Angeles County–University of Southern California (LAC-USC) Women's and Children's Hospital from 1986 to 1993.[2] The hospital is located in East L.A., the largest Mexican barrio in metropolitan Los Angeles, and serves primarily Latina (about 90%), low-income, or indigent women from throughout Los Angeles County.

Case 1:  "G1 P1 SAB 0 TAB 0, 17-yr.-old, r/o herpes" [first pregnancy and birth, no spontaneous or therapeutic abortions, 17-year-old, rule out herpes]

Case 2:  "G1 P1 SAB 0 TAB 0, 14-yr.-old, possible rape" [first pregnancy and birth, 14-year-old, may have been raped during illegal border crossing]

Case 3:  "G3 P2 SAB 1 TAB 0, 16-yr.-old, Spanish, wants IUD, straight from the *ranchito*" [third pregnancy, second birth, one spontaneous abortion, 16-year-old, Spanish speaking, wants to use an intrauterine device for contraception, recently arrived in the United States from a rural area in Mexico]

Case 4:  "G5 P1 SAB 0 TAB 4, 16-yr.-old, *chola*, needs *very special counseling*" [fifth pregnancy, one birth, four therapeutic abortions, uses abortion as her method of contraception]

Case 5:  "Miami Vice"

Case 6:  "G1 P0 SAB 1 TAB 0, 15-yr.-old, wants to get pregnant right away"

Case 7:  "The Burning Bed"

Case 8:  "Fetal demise, refer to Jorge (the high-risk case manager)"

Case 9:  "María, José y Jesús"

Case 10:  "María González"

We referred to the teen mothers served in the clinic by their "disease" just like the "insensitive" physicians did. It was shorthand, a way to signal immediately who we meant, and a way to keep from crying. Most of them, at least at first, were simply known by their reproductive statistics, their disease, or the type of birth-control method they wanted. There were many chart notes indicating the need to rule out different sexually transmitted diseases, especially herpes and condyloma. Fortunately, there were few "possible rapes," at least those known to us. One "possible rape" delivered her infant at home, stabbed it multiple times, and dumped it in a dumpster. The infant was discovered by a passerby but died in the hospital. The mother was already under custody of juvenile authorities and chained to her hospital bed when we interviewed her. Another was raped crossing the border. A more common story, however, was sexual abuse by an adult male living in the household—a stepfather, a mother's boyfriend, an uncle, or a cousin.

Other shorthand items indicated a constellation of social characteristics useful in counseling and helping the young mothers. "Straight from the *ranchito*" indicated that the teen was a recent immigrant, had a traditional gender-role orientation, spoke only Spanish, and would very likely need help negotiating the American medical and social service system. "Needs very special counseling" was shorthand for noncompliant[3] contraceptors who had repeat, unintended pregnancies and multiple abortions. Repeat abortion is particularly difficult for family-planning providers, because it makes them feel as if they have failed the client. "*Chola*," a slang term that refers to youth who identify with the Latino gang culture by dress, behavior, and action (Harris 1988), indicated a possibly gang-involved lifestyle. It alerted us to screen for sexually transmitted infections (STIs), drug use, and other risk behaviors. "SABs [spontaneous abortions or miscarriages] and fetal demises" were among the hardest emotionally. We felt the pain of the mothers' loss, yet we also felt that since they were so young, in the long run this might have been the best outcome—*como Dios quiere* (as God wills). Most of the teens who had experienced fetal loss wanted to get pregnant again right away.

A few cases whose stories were especially horrible were given nicknames for quick reference. "Miami Vice" ran away from home to Miami with a man who was later convicted for murder. They both sold cocaine along the way. "The Burning Bed" was a young mother who was being brutally abused by her partner but would not leave. We referred to her using the title of a (then) new made-for-TV movie about spouse abuse starring Farrah Fawcett. "María, José y Jesús" lived in a barn at the race track. We gave them the names of the Holy Family of Christianity, the child living in the stable.

The black humor came naturally, as it does to people in any difficult, stressful, or impossible situation. It helped to insulate "us" from the horrors of the reality of life for "them," these young women we were trying to help. I understand physicians and other clinicians better now, the way they talk about the "hysterectomy in [room] 25" or the "broken leg in the ER [Emergency Room]." It's a shorthand, but it also distances the provider from the patient. It allowed us to offer help and understanding, but it also gave us the ability to detach ourselves emotionally and avoid becoming overwhelmed by their problems.

"María González" was our first HIV-positive case, before the days when the red charts (signifying HIV-positive clients) made up an increasing proportion of the client caseload. We never called her "AIDS" or anything like that. She was known by her own name, a fictitious one here. I think it was impossible for us to joke about her. I met her one day in the summer when I'd gone down to the clinic to abstract some medical records for the project evaluation. María was one of the teens we were hiring with a small grant we'd received from the Los Angeles Women's Foundation to train teen mothers in basic job skills. Of course I'd followed her case, read her medical record, and talked many times with the counselors about her, but the instant I was introduced to her I understood the heterosexual spread of AIDS. She looked like a completely normal, healthy, beautiful young woman poised at the beginning of a life of endless possibilities, not like someone whose blood contained a virus that would lead to almost certain death.[4] What did I expect, that somehow I would be able to tell by looking that a person was HIV infected? It was impossible at that moment to think that in ten years she would probably be dead, as would her boyfriend, who was also HIV positive and was the likely source of her infection. He was a drug dealer and an intravenous drug user. (In January 1996 as I write these words almost eight years later, María's health has declined to the point that death is imminent. She will leave behind her child, who was not infected. Meanwhile, Tina, another HIV-infected young mother, who is herself currently healthy, watches her toddler die of AIDS.)

Over time we became somewhat immune to the hardship stories. Every teen had one. Indeed, we used to sit around and joke about how we had opened Pandora's box, as Blanca the head counselor called it, and were watching first the beautiful and then the ugly things fly out. My metaphor for this is a scene from Steven Spielberg's 1981 film, *Raiders of the Lost Ark*, in which the French archeologist opens the Ark of the Covenant and the Nazis look on, seeing first beauty and then evil, and they die grisly deaths while Dr. Jones and the heroine look away and thus are saved. We must be aware but must not look (i.e., feel too deeply) lest we be consumed. Yet helping young mothers requires delving more deeply into their life circumstances than is usually necessary for standard clinical care. The hardships were just part of the lives of the population served. We learned to expect small victories and be happy with them.

Most of my formal presentations and prior publications on Latina adolescent childbearing have been based on the quantitative evaluation of the efficacy of family-planning case management in the prevention of repeat pregnancy. In this book, I want to look at the problem of teenage pregnancy and childbearing from a more personal and holistic perspective, as observed through my own eyes, through the eyes of the teen mothers, and through those of the counselors in the family-planning clinic who are the *alma y corazón* (heart and soul) of the intervention efforts described here. I was a participant-observer in the anthropological sense, since my role was that of public health researcher, grant writer, and evaluator. What I have learned through ten years of involvement in family planning for Latina adolescents is what I knew all along: that there are many sides to the same story, and each must be considered in order to understand the problem.

I was inspired to write this book by the apparent differences between the Latina teens with whom I had been working and the teens described in the literature on teenage pregnancy among African American and white populations in the United States. This literature characterizes teen pregnancy and childbearing as a medical and sociological problem with many adverse physical, emotional, developmental, and socioeconomic outcomes (Hatcher et al. 1989). What I began noticing was that most of the young Latinas in our project had relatively good birth outcomes despite poor prenatal care, many had planned their pregnancies, and they also had a high level of social support from partners and family. This suggested a rather different picture of teenage pregnancy among this particular population of Latina teens in East L.A.

Additionally, I began to become aware of a mismatch between the needs of the young mothers and the medical interventions and prevention strategies used in the program. Preventing repeat pregnancy and promoting return to school—major goals of most programs—may actually be irrelevant for many Latina teens, particularly those who are recent immigrants.

This is reminiscent of the many situations of culture contact between the developed and less-developed countries and the possible conflicts with and misunderstandings of the Western biomedical system described by anthropologists in developing countries (see McElroy and Townsend 1989 or Paul 1955 for an overview of this problem). The phenomenon is becoming increasingly common within the United States as more and more diverse ethnic and cultural groups make a permanent home here. The history of the diffusion of modern methods of contraception throughout the world is a relevant example. Modern methods of contraception were encouraged for use in the rural areas of many countries where initially there was little demand for them. Issues intertwined with culture and subsistence patterns, including gender roles, the economic utility of children in rural agrarian societies, the need for high fertility to hedge against high infant and child mortality, the need for children to support you in your old age, and the ritual importance of male children in some societies, as well as other factors, all played a significant role in thwarting the efforts at population control, a problem defined by Western science and society.

As in the case of family planning abroad, the trend toward the medicalization of domestic social problems that have a medical component (e.g., adolescent pregnancy, drug use, violence, child abuse, homelessness) further complicates the picture (see Lupton 1994). Medicalization results in the infusion of the "problem" with the cultural and moral values of those who "treat" the "ill," the health care practitioners. According to Kunitz (1989), the health profession, which still consists largely of members of the dominant middle-class white society, is increasingly able to define morality *via* its treatment of these social problems in a medical setting. What this means is that adolescent pregnancy and childbearing have come to be defined as aberrant behaviors because they come before both the medically and socially sanctioned decades of optimal childbearing in American society (i.e., age 20–35). Thus, intervention programs are directed at prevention of early childbearing and attempt to help young mothers "get back on track" with their education, molding them toward middle-class ideals.

In this book I explore the hypothesis that teenage pregnancy among Latinas may be different than that among African American and white American teenagers because of different normative cultural expectations for young women, particularly for those who have recently arrived in the United States and therefore are less acculturated to American society. I draw on ten years of research and clinical experience with Latina teen mothers to describe the social context of teenage pregnancy. The data were collected using informal structured interviews, key informant interviewing, systematic data collection techniques (Bernard 1994; Weller and Romney 1988), and participant observation in the clinic setting. The data come from four sources:

1. two face-to-face surveys of teen mothers aged 17 and under who delivered at the hospital: 1,017 in 1986–1987 and 1,293 in 1992–1994;
2. a longitudinal study of 173 Latina teen mothers who participated in the Teen Project, a clinic-based repeat-pregnancy prevention project, between April 1989 and December 1991;

3. qualitative interviews with Latina teens and family-planning providers (28 teens, 13 providers) about attitudes toward contraceptive methods, life events, and women's roles in 1992;
4. interviews and conversations with project staff, teen mothers, and clinic providers between 1985 and 1995.

These data are used to explore the impact of level of acculturation on the patterning of teen pregnancy in this group and to describe how the cultural patterning of reproductive behavior influences the interaction of these Latina teen mothers with an intervention program designed by middle-class health care professionals. It appears that such projects, while well intentioned, essentially miss the point by assuming that teen pregnancy is not a rational choice and must certainly be maladaptive rather than being self-enhancing, even beneficial, under existing socioeconomic and political circumstances. There is an increasing recognition among researchers that early childbearing may be a rational choice in the face of extremely bleak life options (Burton 1990; Geronimus and Korenman 1993; Luker 1991, 1996; Zabin and Hayward 1993).

In order to describe the sociocultural context of teenage pregnancy in this group, I use the triangulation method described by Scrimshaw and Hurtado (1987), in which quantitative data (surveys, medical records) and qualitative data (interviews and observations) are used to enhance, supplement, and check one another in the interpretation of the results. What is so frequently lacking in sociological or medical accounts of teenage pregnancy is the qualitative perspective that reveals the reasons for teens' behavior. This side of the story is needed to make sense of quantitative results. Quantitative data, on the other hand, provide a measure of assurance that interpretations based on qualitative data are representative of the group under study, thus mitigating the major criticism leveled at qualitative research. The triangulation approach takes advantage of the best of both worlds to provide a deeper understanding of the problem.

The subject under study is complex and plays itself out differently for different individuals and subgroups: the married immigrant teen; the unmarried *chola;* the victim of sexual abuse; or the physically abused teen who remains in the relationship for economic reasons. In order to prevent or delay repeat pregnancy, which was a goal both of the prevention project and of almost all of the participants, the project attempted to facilitate contraceptive use. To increase compliance with the contraceptive regimen, it was necessary to understand more about these young women's lives to help them overcome obstacles to contraceptive use. By asking about their lives and offering to help in any way possible, we opened Pandora's box. The contents of that box are what I hope to communicate in this book. By understanding individual motivations and the circumstances related to teen childbearing, and then relating them to a sociocultural system or environment, we begin to understand teenage pregnancy as it is lived in social and cultural context. I hope this work will contribute to a better understanding of the fertility behavior of Latina adolescents and the interface between Latina teenage mothers and the medically oriented programs designed to help them.

In the following chapters, I describe the characteristics of Latina teen mothers in East L.A. and a clinic-based project that tried to help them. Chapter 2 provides a broader context for the book, discussing the problem of teenage pregnancy in America, providing an overview of Latino cultural attitudes and values relevant to an understanding of teenage pregnancy and childbearing, and providing an overview of research on Latino adolescent sexual and reproductive behavior in the United States. Chapters 3 and 4 describe the history of the Teen Project, the research methods and procedures, and the research setting. Chapter 5 describes the Latina teen mothers and the social context of pregnancy and motherhood: the relationship to the baby's father, living arrangements, social support, whether the pregnancy was intended, school status, plans and goals, and attitudes toward women's roles. Chapters 6 through 8 address issues of health care utilization and outcomes: Chapter 6 discusses prenatal care and birth outcome; Chapter 7 describes the evaluation of the Teen Project and discusses reasons for the limited impact of the project in preventing repeat pregnancy; and Chapter 8 discusses contraceptive use patterns and looks at the structural and cultural barriers to contraceptive use and pregnancy prevention. Throughout these chapters, I discuss how acculturation affects life options among these young women. I use statistical methods, case studies, and interviews to portray adolescent motherhood for this group and to identify the dominant pathways leading to motherhood in this population. I also discuss how social and cultural norms and the realities of everyday life in East L.A. tend to support adolescent motherhood. In the final chapter, I discuss implications of the study for prevention and intervention efforts and for understanding the limitations of current prevention strategies.

It is my hope that this book will lead to an understanding of how adolescent pregnancy and childbearing fit into the fabric of social and cultural life in this particular Latino population. As a public health professional I have been involved in the design and implementation of numerous prevention and intervention projects, from school-based clinics to contraceptive case management for postpartum teen mothers, all of which have had only limited impact on adolescent pregnancy. In exasperation at the failure of the interventions I had been taught would work and the recent documentation of their limited impact (Furstenberg et al. 1987; Luker 1991, 1996; Polit

1989; Polit and Kahn 1985; Zabin and Hayward 1993), I decided I needed to understand more about the social process of becoming a teen mother. This book is the result. The message it holds for health providers is the need for intervention strategies based on an understanding of the context of adolescent motherhood in all its variety.

CHAPTER TWO

# Culture, Norms, and Adolescent Childbearing

## The Problem of
## Adolescent Pregnancy in America

In the 1990s, over half of the 15- to 19-year-olds in the United States are sexually active. By age 20, 75% of females and 80% of males have had intercourse, most premaritally. Trends over the last twenty years have moved toward an earlier age at initiation of sexual intercourse and an increase in the number of sex partners among adolescents. Although contraceptive use has increased, especially the use of condoms, pregnancy rates have hardly changed at all. One in ten teenagers becomes pregnant in the United States every year, a rate much higher than that of any other Western industrialized country. Of the estimated one million teen pregnancies each year, over 80% are unintended. Half result in a live birth, about 40% end in therapeutic abortion, and most of the remainder in miscarriage (Braverman and Strasburger 1993). As Zabin and Hayward (1993) explain, there are really two problems of adolescent pregnancy: one is unprotected sexual activity leading to pregnancy and abortion among middle- and upper-class teens; the other is unprotected intercourse leading to pregnancy and childbearing among poor, inner-city youth, many of whom welcome, or are at least ambivalent about, becoming a mother.

When President Clinton declared war on adolescent pregnancy in January 1995 and continued the battle in January 1996, he brought the "problem" of teenage childbearing back into the consciousness of the American public. The president's revival of the teenage motherhood problem and the Republican response of attempting to deny welfare to teen mothers are only the latest skirmishes in the twenty-year debate and public concern about how to reverse the trends in the sexual behavior of American teens (Hayes 1987; Nathanson 1991; Zabin and Hayward 1993).

Interest in teenage childbearing probably began with the influential 1976 publication of the Alan Guttmacher Institute's *Eleven Million Teenagers: What Can Be Done about the Epidemic of Adolescent Pregnancies in the United States*. With this publication, teenage pregnancy was elevated to epidemic status, requiring swift measures to control its spread. But was there really an epidemic?

In the early 1980s, Vinovskis (1981) and Davis (1980) were among the first to point out that the problem of adolescent pregnancy in the United States was really an economic and moral problem associated with changes in adolescent fertility patterns beginning in the 1960s. These changes included increasing rates of premarital sexual activity among adolescents, their use of contraception and abortion, increasing rates of illegitimate births, and the greater public cost borne by society for children of unmarried teen parents. Although the overall teenage fertility rate has been steadily declining since the 1950s, the increase in illegitimate births to teens, from 15% in 1960 to 31% in 1970 to 60% in 1987 (Nathanson 1991), was so dramatic that Kingsley Davis was prompted to write: "The only soaring aspect of teenage fertility is illegitimate fertility . . ." (1980, 324). Along with this change in illegitimate birth rates there was also a significant change in adoption patterns. In the 1960s, 90% of illegitimate children born to teenage mothers were relinquished for adoption. In the 1980s, 96% of single teen mothers kept and raised their children themselves, making the problem much more visible (Alan Guttmacher Institute 1981; Nathanson 1991; Vinovskis 1981). Moreover, with the 1973 legalization of abortion after *Roe v. Wade*, increasing numbers of teens chose to abort. The escalation of violence against abortion providers, witnessed over the last decade, attests to the deep cleavage in moral values surrounding sexuality and abortion in the United States today.

Thus, it was a change in adolescent fertility patterns—a change that was much more dramatic among white adolescents—and the social and economic implications of this change, rather than increasing teenage birth rates, that was at the core of the public concern about teenage pregnancy. The epidemic was an epidemic of illegitimate births. As Nathanson notes: "By eschewing marriage and adoption as means of concealment, adolescent women in general, and white women in particular, substantially increased the visibility of reproductive patterns in conflict with traditional social norms" (1991, 30). For many Americans, then, morality is the issue. The double transgression of out-of-time and out-of-wedlock childbearing challenges the core values of the middle class and becomes one of the major issues in the debate about adolescent childbearing. Thus, the agenda driving public attention to the adolescent pregnancy problem is the social control of female adolescent sexuality.

The other major issue of concern to Americans is the public burden of support for the multitude of negative medical and social outcomes associated with adolescent childbearing. This issue, embodied in Aid to Families with Dependent Children (AFDC), Medicaid, and other welfare programs, has achieved increasing attention from politicians, especially conservatives, throughout the 1980s and 1990s, culminating in the recent restructuring, some might say dismantling, of the welfare system in this country.

### Medical Risks of Teen Childbearing

Except for the very youngest, teenage mothers are not medically at risk because of age alone. Rather they are at risk because of other factors such as poor prenatal care, poor nutrition, and lifestyle factors including violence and substance use (Baldwin and Cain 1980; Menken 1981). Early studies found greater rates of medical complications such as anemia, pregnancy-induced hypertension, toxemia, prematurity, and perinatal and maternal mortality among adolescents than among older women (Gordon et al. 1979; Graham 1981). Although recent data suggest that adolescents can fare as well as or better than adult women if they have good prenatal care, adolescents in contemporary American society are less likely than adults to receive prenatal care and more likely to initiate it later in the pregnancy when they do receive care (Brindis and Jeremy 1988; Brown 1988; Rothenberg and Varga 1981; Singh et al. 1985). Reasons for inadequate prenatal care among adolescents include not recognizing and/or concealing pregnancy, not realizing the importance and availability of prenatal care, and not being able to afford care. Thus, even though they might have a slight biological advantage over older women, their less adequate use of prenatal care undermines that advantage.

Because of this, serious medical complications are still associated with adolescent childbearing. These include low birth weight, toxemia (pre-eclampsia or eclampsia), and prematurity—outcomes also associated with poor prenatal care (Gordon et al. 1979; Graham 1981; Wallace et al. 1988). In addition, the children of teen parents are at greater risk of morbidity and mortality than children of older parents (Gordon et al. 1979).

### Social and Economic Risks

If teens received comprehensive prenatal care services, most of the medical problems associated with adolescent childbearing could be avoided. The social and economic risks, however, may be less easy to ameliorate than the medical ones. In comparison to women who wait until their twenties to begin childbearing, teen mothers complete fewer years of formal education, have lower socioeconomic status, are more likely to be dependent on welfare, have higher divorce rates, have higher total completed fertility and more closely spaced births, have children with lower cognitive development, and are more likely to abuse their own children (Baldwin and Cain 1980; Card 1981; Card and Wise 1978; Dryfoos 1982; Hatcher et al. 1981, 1989; Hayes 1987; Mott and Marsiglio 1985; Zabin and Hayward 1993). More recent work suggests a delayed effect of early birth on child abuse such that older children rather than infants are the targets of abuse and neglect (Miller and Moore 1990). In addition, teen mothers have an elevated rate of suicide compared to other adolescents (Hatcher et al. 1981). Recent studies suggest that they are also more likely than nonmothers to have a history of sexual abuse (Berenson et al. 1992; Boyer and Fine 1992; Parker et al. 1993).

### Partners of Teen Mothers: Forgotten Males

There has been very little research on the partners of teens who become pregnant, perhaps because of the difficulty of gaining access to the population. Less than one-quarter (23%) of the fathers of babies born to teenagers are teens themselves, and studies suggest they represent a wide age range, from 15 to 69 (Hardy 1988). Among teen mothers aged 15 to 17, more than half of the fathers are 20 years of age or older; 25% of them are three to five years and 19% are more than six years older than the teen mother (Landry and Forrest 1995). As these authors note, such wide gaps in age and the corresponding differences in life experience and power within the relationship suggest the possibility of sexual abuse or, at the very least, pressure. Despite the fact that most of the fathers involved are not themselves teenagers, most research has focused on adolescent fathers and suggests that they suffer similar disadvantages with respect to socioeconomic variables as do teenage mothers (Card and Wise 1978). Several studies also suggest that, contrary to popular opinion, many teen fathers remain involved with their children, at least in the short term, even if the couple does not marry. Problems facing the adolescent father include those related to his role as provider and to difficulties in his relationship to the mother of the child and to her family (Barret and Robinson 1982a, 1982b; Hendricks and Montgomery 1983; Pleck et al. 1993; Zayas et al. 1987). Marsiglio (1993) found that among 15- to 19-year-old males in his nationally representative sample, low socioeconomic status was related to less frequent contraceptive use and positive attitudes toward unplanned pregnancy. Aside from their ages, little is known regarding the bulk of the progenitors who are adult men.

### Children of Teen Mothers

The children of teen mothers are likely to be economically and developmentally disadvantaged and to do more poorly in school. Studies of cognitive development have shown that children of young mothers fare less well than children of older mothers, although the difference is small. With respect to cognitive development, however, maternal age has less explanatory power than socioeconomic status (Hatcher et al. 1989). There is also some evidence to suggest that young mothers are less able to respond appropriately to the developmental needs of their children (Hardy 1982; Miller and Moore 1990). Children of teenage mothers also tend to repeat the cycle of early childbearing, early marriage, and higher fertility of their parents, and these adverse social outcomes are more likely if the young mother raises her child(ren) alone without the support of their father or her own parents (Baldwin and Cain 1980; Dryfoos 1982; Miller and Moore 1990).

Clearly, then, there is ample evidence that teenage childbearing and child-rearing are not optimal, at least not under current social and economic conditions in the United States. The adverse social, economic, and medical outcomes for teen mothers, fathers, and their children are serious and justify public concern. They are also expensive.

### Public Cost

In the 1980s, much attention was devoted to assessing the public cost of teenage mothers and their children. In 1985, in California alone, it was estimated that over $3 billion was spent on families that were begun when the mother was a teenager (Brindis and Jeremy 1988). Nationwide in 1988 an estimated $20 billion was spent by U.S. taxpayers to support families begun when the mother was a teenager (Center for Population Options 1989; Burt 1986). Thus, the burden of public support for teen mothers and their children through welfare, Medicaid, and other programs for poor women and children is considerable.

### A Minority Issue?

Another important aspect of the adolescent pregnancy problem is its association with minority status.[1] Numerous studies have shown that adolescent childbearing, though not pregnancy, is associated with minority status, lower socioeconomic level, school failure and school dropout, and residence in a single-female–headed household—all factors that may be interrelated (Cooksey 1990; Dryfoos 1982; Furstenberg et al. 1987; Marini 1978, 1984; Rindfuss et al. 1984; Upchurch and McCarthy 1990; Zabin and Hayward 1993). Although in terms of absolute numbers the majority of teen births are to whites (because they make up a majority of the population), proportionately more minority youths have babies while they are teenagers. In 1990, the birth rate to 15- to 19-year-olds was 116.2 per thousand for African Americans, 100.3 for Latinas, and 45.2 for whites (*MMWR* 1993).

Moreover, most of the studies of adolescent childbearing and most of the media attention to the problem has focused on African Americans to the extent that many Americans perceive it to be an African American problem. Thus, as Nathanson notes: "In recent years, as moral and fiscal conservatives have gained increasing ascendance in domestic policy–making circles, adolescent pregnancy itself has become redefined as a 'black' problem" (1991, 35). Although birth rates to Latina teens are also high, only in the last decade have researchers paid attention to reproductive trends among Latina youth. The lack of data about Latina teen childbearing prior to the late 1980s lowered the visibility of the magnitude of the problem among Latinas, and consequently Latina teens were neglected by health and social service providers and policymakers (Fennelly 1993).

Politically, then, adolescent pregnancy is a costly health and social problem. It pits conservatives against liberals in the battle over welfare, abortion, morality, and the social control of female sexuality, privileging middle-class norms and values. Research, prevention efforts, and intervention programs have been aimed at changing individual behavior to bring it in line with middle-class American norms. But exactly what are these norms and how do they affect behavior?

## Norms and Behavior

Jencks (1990) has described two middle-class norms for childbearing: (1) people should not have children until they are in their twenties, and (2) they should try to avoid having children out of wedlock. If they do have children while unmarried, however, they should be able to support them economically. Middle-class children are expected first to finish high school and, increasingly, to complete college (ages 18–25) in order to get a well-paying, rewarding job. Only then should they marry (ages 20–30) and have children (commencing 1–2 years after marriage), but only if they can provide for them. Norms proscribing premarital sex and abortion are still held by many Americans, although in the 1990s premarital sexual experience is normative behavior and abortion is legal if not always accessible (Blum 1991; Miller and Moore 1990; Newcomer and Baldwin 1992).

Although most would recognize the American script described above as common cultural knowledge, empirical demonstration of its validity is difficult. This stems from the fact that there are different ways in which normative behavior is conceptualized. Indeed, a major problem in research on the normative ordering of life events is that the term itself is ambiguous.

On the one hand, normative behavior can be empirically based, reflecting actual population trends. Sociology and demography have described trends in reproductive events statistically, and, as we shall see, the middle-class script suggested above is reflected in the overall timing of these events in the American population. In this literature, norms are based on statistical population trends (i.e., mean, median, or modal age at transition), making the norm equivalent to what actually happens to most people.

On the other hand, there is the more value-laden sense in which normative order is used to imply the appropriate order in which events "should" take place, as in Jencks's characterization of middle-class childbearing norms. In this sense, normative order takes into consideration both moral prescriptions for timing of sex, marriage, and children (e.g., the Judeo-Christian imperative of marriage before intercourse and childbearing) and class-based norms for level of education and type of occupation that, in turn, delay the appropriate age for reproductive events into the twenties and sometimes the thirties. The extent to which the idealized order and actual behavior overlap can be considered a measure of cultural consensus on life-course norms.

## Timing of Transition Events

Transition events are singular events in the life of an individual that signal change from one social status to another (e.g., high school graduation, marriage, first birth). Quantitative data on the timing of transition events among women in the United States provide empirical evidence for the saliency of the American script described earlier (see Table 2.1). In a recent article, Forrest (1993) presents data on age at reproductive transition events (i.e., intercourse, pregnancy, cohabitation/marriage, first birth) for a nationally representative sample of women. As seen in Table 2.1, the median age (age by which half of the women in the sample completed the event) at marriage is 24.3 and comes after the normative age for school completion in the United States (18 for high school, 22–23 for college), and the age at first birth comes two years after marriage. The data also suggest, however, that this pattern is most applicable to white women and to women at or above 200% of poverty.[2]

Among white women, most fulfill the normative middle-class pattern of marriage prior to having their first child, but among Latina and African American women the trend is reversed, and the age at first birth is quite a bit younger (about four years) than it is among whites. The similarity between the pattern among Latina and African American women and among women below 200% of poverty suggests that, at least in part, the pattern among minority women is likely to be heavily influenced by socioeconomic class. Unfortunately, Forrest did not analyze her data by poverty status

Table 2.1.    Median Age at Transition Events for American Women in 1988

| Event | Ethnicity | | | | % of Poverty | |
| | All | White | African American | Latina | <200% | >200% |
|---|---|---|---|---|---|---|
| Intercourse | 17.4 | 17.6 | 16.6 | 17.7 | 17.2 | 17.6 |
| Pregnancy | 21.3 | 22.0 | 19.3 | 20.6 | 20.4 | 22.1 |
| Cohabitation or Marriage | 22.0 | 21.8 | 21.0 | 21.8 | 22.0 | 22.0 |
| Marriage | 24.3 | 23.8 | 28.3 | 23.9 | 24.7 | 24.0 |
| First Birth | 26.0 | 26.7 | 22.5 | 22.7 | 23.0 | 28.1 |

*Source:* Forrest 1993:107

within race/ethnic groups, but overall levels of poverty are known to be higher among minority women.

Data on level of education completed also suggest that, as with reproductive events, different norms (i.e., different actual behavior) may be operative. By age 25, the median years of education completed by both African Americans and whites is 12.0 years, for those of Mexican heritage 9.1 years (11.7 for U.S.-born and 6.1 for foreign-born), and for Central and South Americans 11.7 years (12.4 for U.S.-born and 11.7 for foreign-born; Bean and Tienda 1987). Thus, overall, normative education completed by those of Mexican origin (the largest Latino group in the United States) is quite a bit lower than that for other groups, but this is mediated to a large degree by generation (e.g., first generation is foreign-born, second generation is U.S.-born with one or more parents foreign-born, etc.) in the United States.

In sum, these data suggest rather different patterns of behavior by race, ethnicity, and social class. Statistical trends among whites tend to mirror the middle-class American cultural script described earlier and to adhere to moral (childbearing after marriage) and class (completion of at least high school before marriage and childbearing) considerations of appropriate behavior. Among Latinas and African American women, however, we see an alternate normative (i.e., actual) course in which childbearing tends to occur much earlier and before marriage. Finally, among Latinos, educational achievement norms are lower than those of other groups. Reproductive patterns, however, appear to be mediated by socioeconomic status, and education among Latinos appears to be mediated by area of origin and generation in the United States. Thus, the middle-class American script does not necessarily apply to Americans of different social class, race, culture, or ethnicity. Not only is the timing of events earlier, but the sequencing of events is different. To what extent are these alternate life-course patterns reflected in idealized norms?

### Alternate Life-Course Strategies?

Do adolescent mothers from any racial or ethnic group share the middle-class script that defines their own behavior as aberrant? If they do share the script, why are they unable to make their lives conform to the ideal? Or, is it simply irrelevant to their lives? What is the relationship between ideal norms and actual behavior? Does one cause the other or are they mutually reinforcing? These are important questions that have only recently begun to receive the attention of researchers.

A few studies suggest that alternate reproductive strategies are recognized as normative among defined groups of African Americans (Burton 1990; Franklin 1988). Burton (1990) described norms for rural, low-income, multigenerational African American families in which women bore children in early adolescence, and the children were then raised by their grandmothers. This pattern was perceived by members of the culture as normative. Altering it would deny a generation of women the chance to be mothers, a strong deterrent to change in individual behavior for young teens. In a similar vein, other researchers have begun to pose the possibility that early childbearing may be a rational choice in the face of extremely bleak life options (Burton 1990; Geronimus and Korenman 1993; Luker 1991, 1996; Zabin and Hayward 1993). Moreover, it is likely, with the tremendous changes in family structure and high divorce rates in the United States over the past two decades, that changes in what is considered normative may already have occurred among younger cohorts who have, thus far, not reached positions of political power necessary to assert the hegemony of their viewpoint (see Cooksey 1990; Luker 1991, 1996; Nathanson 1991).[3]

The assumptions about normative behavior underlying most adolescent childbearing prevention and intervention programs, however, often ignore even the possibility of alternative, more positive interpretations of early childbearing. Twenty years of primary prevention efforts (to prevent or delay initiation of sexual intercourse or, failing that, to prevent pregnancy and sexually transmitted diseases through contraception and safe-sex practices) and secondary prevention efforts (to ameliorate the adverse effects of teen-age childbearing and prevent repeat pregnancy) have met with only limited success (Braverman and Strasburger 1993; Frost and Forrest 1995; Furstenberg 1976; Furstenberg et al. 1987; Luker 1991; Polit 1989; Polit and Kahn 1985). Nor have they been able to alter the lack of opportunities and harsh economic realities facing minority populations and poor women and children of all races in the United States.

## Are Middle-Class Programs Relevant to Poor Teen Mothers?

The medical interventions for adolescent pregnancy in the United States are directed toward good ends: the birth of a healthy infant, a healthy mother, and the provision of contraceptive methods to prevent repeat pregnancies among adolescent mothers. The social interventions that often take place within clinical medical settings, however, are directed toward the American script for normative life events: school, work, and economic self-sufficiency. Compliance is largely dependent on acceptance of the dominant culture's negative interpretation of adolescent pregnancy and childbearing and the teen mothers' ability to access pertinent resources (i.e., education, employment). The underlying causes of early childbearing, however, appear to be poverty and lack of access to those very resources of education and employment (see Luker 1996). Lack of opportunity fosters early and out-of-wedlock childbearing. Over time, behavioral norms may become reflected in cultural scripts that support a normative life course that deviates from the ideal, and actual, middle-class life course. Behavior and norms, then, interact to perpetuate these alternative childbearing patterns intergenerationally.

Neither poverty nor values can be addressed effectively in short-term, often clinically based, programs. Thus, most programs have failed to be effective in the prevention and amelioration of teenage childbearing because, as Luker (1991, 1996) has suggested, they assume that teen pregnancy is an individual problem that can be treated outside the social and cultural context of young mothers' lives. Indeed, it is probable that the failure of current programs to have more than a limited impact on the larger adolescent sexuality and pregnancy problem stems from social policy that focuses on individual change and grossly underestimates the powerful social, cultural, and economic forces that favor teenage motherhood among women of color and lower socioeconomic status.

## Culture and Behavior: An Anthropological Perspective

Lucille Newman (1978) was one of the first anthropologists to suggest that cultural norms for transition events are implicit guides for individual behavior. She pointed out that people in any society have a definite idea about the ideal order and timing of major life events such as school, work, marriage, and children, and that these "cultural scripts" can be quite different for different cultures. Cultural scripts can have a strong influence on fertility patterns because they set standards, customs, and norms for such intermediate fertility variables as age at union formation and childbearing (Bongaarts 1982; Davis and Blake 1956). Thus, cultural scripts can be seen both as important guides for personal behavior at one level, and as explanations of particular fertility patterns at a more abstract level.

Anthropologists, like Newman, would attribute overriding importance to the way in which social and cultural norms shape sexual behavior. Yet, variation in norms, or cultural scripts, has only recently come to be seriously addressed in research on teen pregnancy in the United States. This is largely due to the fact that most of the research and the resulting literature on adolescent childbearing has been generated by health practitioners, health researchers, and social scientists who are themselves embedded in their own cultural perspective. Moreover, they are not trained to give primacy to culture as an independent variable. Hence, in this sense, considerations of culture and a larger concern with the importance of historical context are largely absent from the bulk of work on teen pregnancy in other disciplines. Missing, in particular, is the sense of the historical recency of the current pattern of delayed family formation in the United States and the sense that this pattern is not the only alternative, nor indeed even the most common pattern cross-culturally (Eisenberg 1984). Rather, it is embedded in the current cultural, political, ideological, moral, and socioeconomic structures of American society. Moreover, as we have already seen, there are distinct differences in reproductive and educational behavior in the United States by ethnicity and socioeconomic status. These patterns are currently denied normative status by the larger society, but in terms of understanding adolescent pregnancy, we might do better if we considered them as cultural scripts expressing and shaping subcultural (i.e., race, ethnic, and class) differences in the timing of life-course events (Franklin 1988).

There is a wealth of anthropological information that documents a wide range of cultural scripts for sexual behavior and childbearing (Ford 1964; Ford and Beach 1951; Jordan 1978; Kay 1982; Lancaster and Hamburg 1986; Mead and Newton 1967; Miller and Newman 1978; Newman 1985; Newton 1967). In most of the world, women still achieve adult status largely through marriage and motherhood in the middle (15–17) to late (18–19) teenage years (Lancaster and Hamburg 1986). This is certainly the pattern in many areas of Latin America today, as it was in rural American society prior to World War II.

In much of Latin America, especially in rural areas, courting begins about age 15 and proceeds to marriage or informal union formation between ages 16 and 18. Premarital intercourse is variously tolerated, and pregnancy may or may not trigger union formation depending on ethnic identity, religiosity, and social-class variables. While the Latin American middle- and upper-class ideal is premarital chastity prior to marriage in the Catholic Church, the reality among the working classes is often premarital pregnancy followed by informal union, which is sometimes legitimated, sooner or later, by formal marriage. This pattern is common among the lower classes and rural populations who make up the bulk of Latin American society. As in American society, normative ideals can exist that have little consistency with normative behavior. It is likely that Latina adolescents in the United States will be affected by both the ideal norms for behavior and the actual behavior patterns in both the United States and their country of origin or ethnic heritage.

### The Historical Normalcy of Adolescent Childbearing

Lancaster and Hamburg (1986) as well as others (Davis 1980; Vinovskis 1981) remind us that adolescent childbearing was the norm throughout human history when menarche occurred much later and marriage much earlier than in the industrialized countries today. Changes in these biosocial factors have contributed to the adolescent pregnancy problem in the United States. With menarche currently around age 12, there is a very long period, eight or more years, during which American adolescents are expected to abstain from sexual intercourse or use contraception to prevent an untimely pregnancy. As Whiting et al. (1986) point out, this relatively long period of maidenhood is typical of modern, industrialized countries, but can hardly be characterized as normative for either historical or contemporary human populations living in less-industrialized countries and rural areas. Estimates of the current duration of maidenhood (defined as age at marriage minus age at menarche) for twenty-eight contemporary nations yielded a range of 1.8 years for Bangladesh to 11.8 years for Japan. Whiting et al. go on to describe various maidenhood strategies that, they assert, are attuned to social, technological, and environmental factors. For example, short duration of maidenhood appears to be associated with age at marriage close to age at menarche, an emphasis on high fertility, and a rural agricultural subsistence pattern. They also discuss the role of these intermediate fertility variables (Bongaarts 1982; Davis and Blake 1956) in maintaining various maidenhood strategies.

In contrast to much of human history, the constellation of factors surrounding adolescence in industrialized countries today is unprecedented. These factors include the secular trend toward lower age at menarche during the twentieth century, an increasing age at marriage, and the increased demand for a lengthy period of education necessitated by the employment structure. This results in ". . . the widest separation between biological and social maturation known in human history" (Lancaster and Hamburg 1986, 12; also see Eisenberg 1984). Moreover, the predominance of the nuclear family ideal and the increasing cost of living make adolescent parenthood problematic within the current American socioeconomic system.

### Social Organization and Successful
### Adolescent Childbearing

While adolescent childbearing may be more normative both historically and in other parts of the world than it is in the United States today, it is clear that it requires a particular type of social organization to be successful. Where adolescent childbearing is normative, there are a number of social supports for young families that include extended family households and economic systems in which adolescents are able to function as adults and meet their subsistence needs (Konner and Shostak 1986). Perhaps this type of extended support system combined with intergenerational norms for early childbearing is a key to the persistence of teenage motherhood among African Americans (Burton 1990; Snow 1993; Stack 1974). Might this also be a factor for Latinas? How does culture shape the reproductive behavior of Latina teens?

Latinos, especially Latino immigrants to the United States, may be influenced by normative scripts for transition events that vary from the American script in ways that make adolescent childbearing more culturally acceptable. These differences may be related to the acceptability of lower chronological age at family formation events, or the degree of permissiveness in the actual order of those events.

Since social norms about sexual behavior and family formation are shaped by culture,[4] it is not unreasonable to expect that different cultural and ethnic groups might have different norms about sexual behavior and childbearing that would affect adolescent sexual behavior in those groups. In fact, as previously discussed, there is a wealth of anthropological information that documents a wide range of cultural norms for both sexual behavior and childbearing. Additionally, actual reproductive behavior patterns differ among different racial, ethnic, and class groups in the United States today, although the extent to which those patterns reflect ideal norms for behavior is unknown. Among whites, however, actual behavior patterns reflected idealized norms quite well. Thus, it is reasonable to suspect that cultural values will be important in the patterning of teenage sexual behavior among different ethnic groups in the United States. It is even possible that culture may have an effect beyond that of socioeconomic status, the major factor associated with American adolescent childbearing.

### Fertility and Adult Status

Most cultures, American culture included, see fertility as a sign of adult status and worth. Marriage and motherhood as the hallmarks of adult status for women are amply documented in the anthropological record (Miller and Newman 1978). This may be breaking down in more industrialized countries and in urban areas of the developing world, especially where the feminist movement has facilitated a redefinition of sex roles. However, throughout most of the world, women still achieve adult social status largely through marriage and motherhood, often in the middle (15–17) to late (18–19) teenage years. For example, in much of rural agrarian India, Bangladesh, and Pakistan, women are married shortly after menarche. Marriage is often arranged and brides are expected to be virgins. Pregnancy is expected within the first two years of marriage, and high fertility is prized, since children provide essential labor. In rural agrarian areas of Latin America, the pattern is similar except that young persons are free to choose their own partners. After union formation, pregnancy is eagerly anticipated, and moderately high fertility is encouraged. This same pattern characterized rural American society prior to World War II. In all cases the value systems supporting high fertility patterns and the high value placed on the maternal role tended to persist long after the need for high fertility diminished (i.e., the demographic transition).

For ethnic minorities in contemporary American society, if the role of wife and mother is highly valued in their own culture or early family formation is the rule, early childbearing may make "cultural sense." It may also make economic sense for young women whose chances of achieving the level of education required for meaningful participation in the labor force are poor and for whom there are few other realistic alternatives for achieving adult status. In such cases, marriage, informal union, or welfare may provide the economic resources for adult independence.

## Latino Cultural Values

### Primacy of Motherhood and Marriage

The young Latina mothers who are the subject of this book—whether recent immigrants, more acculturated immigrants with bilingual skills and longer residence in the United States, or U.S.-born—have in common a culture that has been portrayed as idealizing motherhood. Numerous writers have noted that within Latino culture the role of wife and mother is highly respected and considered the pinnacle of success for women (Alvirez 1973; Amaro 1988; Andrade 1980; Esparza 1979; Grebler et al. 1970; Kay 1978; Marin et al. 1981; Martinez 1981; Melville 1980; Molina and Aguirre-Molina 1994; Pavich 1986; Scrimshaw 1978a; Wilkinson 1987; Williams 1990). Williams, in her study of the Mexican American family, describes this traditional, religion-based cultural pattern as follows:

> It was taken for granted that all men and women would marry and have children, and many did so in their teens. This was reinforced by the Catholic Church, where marriage and childbearing are considered to be part of God's plan for human beings. Marriage was vital, for homemaking and the bearing of children were considered the ultimate fulfillment of a woman's life in this world. (Williams 1990, 27)

Bettina Flores, in her self-help book for Latinas, *Chiquita's Cocoon*, corroborates the importance of marriage.

> Marriage is the one thing Latinas look forward to with elation. This is understandable because of their conditioning. *"Cuando te cases . . ."* [italics mine] (When you get married . . .) is a daily sermon throughout their lives. (1990, 46).

In addition, birth control is rarely used before the first birth, which is eagerly awaited by most women (Kay 1978; Shedlin and Hollerbach 1981). Many studies have shown that Latina women tend to enter into marriage and childbearing at earlier ages, and to want and to have more children than whites (Bean and Tienda 1987; Marin et al. 1981; Molina and Aguirre-Molina 1994). Indeed, by age 20, 34% of Latina females are already married (Fennelly 1993). A few authors have suggested that entry into a sexual union may more often be precipitated by pregnancy among Latinos, and that this may even be one of the more common paths to adult roles (Becerra and de Anda 1984; Salazar 1979; Salguero 1984). This is certainly the pattern in rural areas and among lower-class urban populations throughout Latin America.

### Gender-Role Norms and the Family

Most writers on Latino culture stress that family is extremely important to Latinos and that men and women adhere to traditional gender roles to a greater extent than in the dominant culture. These family patterns are reinforced by machismo, respect, and the subordination of younger to older persons (Pavich 1986). Machismo is a constellation of expectations regarding masculinity that include:

> . . . virility, pride, authoritarianism, prowess, courage, honor, respect for others, and provision for the needs of the family. This overcompensa-

tory "machismo" may take the form of fighting, bragging, drinking, and continual seeking of sexual conquests. The Chicano male is traditionally encouraged to be sexually active from his adolescence onward. (1986, 52–53)

On the other hand, Latina women

> have been socialized to value others before themselves . . . From child-hood, girls are taught household duties in preparation for the only roles ultimately expected of them: those of wife and mother. . . . They may have very few friends beyond the extended family, so that their sources of information about life are restricted to those persons who share the same beliefs. With the maternal role most highly valued . . . [in response to overcompensatory machismo] the mother may show the patience, suffering, and forbearance which is characteristic of the "marianisma" role. (Pavich 1986, 53–54)

Although these stereotyped versions of gender behavior are still influential in Latino culture, changes in socioeconomic realities necessitating female labor participation, the emergence of middle- and upper-class Latinos, and exposure to the more egalitarian gender norms of Anglo middle-class culture result in variation in actual gender behavior among Latinos. Some studies suggest that Mexican American women exposed to the feminist movement in the United States have changed their attitudes toward traditional roles only slightly (Wilkinson 1987). Others suggest that there is conflict between Latino males and females regarding traditional gender roles, with males adhering to more traditional role orientations than females, even among those who are more educated (González 1993). Williams indicates that regardless of social class, the husbands in her study continued to wield more power than their wives (Williams 1990). Still others suggest that, in general, acculturation, or more accurately biculturalism, and generation in the United States tend to liberalize gender-role attitudes for both sexes but do not undermine the importance of family (Amaro 1988; González 1993; Hurtado et al. 1992; Kranau et al. 1982; Vega 1990). Thus, gender-role patterns appear to be in flux, with generation, socioeconomic status, and acculturation as important mediating factors.

### Early Marriage and School Leaving

Consistent with the earlier marriage pattern among Latinos, it has been noted that Latino adolescents tend to take on adult roles earlier than whites and that reaching higher levels of schooling tends not to be as important an ideal for Latinos as for African Americans and whites. This is particularly true for Latina females. For example, a sixth-grade education for females is considered a good education in Mexico and may be quite acceptable among the more recently arrived Mexican immigrants in the United States as well (Rosina M. Becerra, personal communication, 1987). This contrasts with the ideal in the United States of at least high school graduation. Thus, early school leaving (prior to pregnancy) may be an important factor contributing to teenage pregnancy in this group and may lead, more or less naturally, to the earlier assumption of the role of wife and/or mother.

Levels of education completed by Latinos in the United States do, in fact, tend to be lower than those for whites or African Americans. The discrepancy is particularly marked for foreign-born individuals (Bean and Tienda 1987; Hayes-Bautista et al. 1988; Hurtado et al. 1992; Molina and Aguirre-Molina 1994). While socioeconomic status is certainly a factor in education level and, overall, Latinos have lower incomes than either African Americans or whites, successive generations of Latinos, in California at least, reach higher levels of schooling, although still below those of African Americans and whites, but college graduates are particularly underrepresented (Hurtado et al. 1992).

Flores illuminates:

> Latinas are barely making it through high school. . . . Poverty, early pregnancy, marriage and the desire to enter the work force are the sources of this problem, according to statisticians. . . . Perhaps Latinas reject education because of their conditioning during their formative years. They are expected to carry heavy loads of work at home. . . . With these motivation killers [housework and sometimes employment] and lack of familial encouragement Latinas have to go it alone . . . more important, at what point in their lives do Latinas begin to reject education? Is it when the kindergarten teacher tells them they may only speak English at school? Or in the fourth grade, when the easy ABC's turn into the more difficult social sciences? Or in junior high, where taking group showers is a requirement? Or maybe, in high school where the temptations of sex, romance and marriage are dominant. . . . [Or when a college student comes home for vacation and says] "My friends and family shunned me and treated me as though I didn't belong anymore." (1990, 34–35)

A study of the impact of pregnancy and childbearing on dropping out of school in the Southwest supports the idea that Latinos may have different values regarding school, entry into marriage, and family responsibilities (Kaplan 1990). Although pregnancy was one of the reasons, and accounted for about one-third of school dropouts, it was not the primary cause of dropout among Latina females. Other factors were also important in the multiple regression analysis performed, including the low education level of Latino males, a high sex ratio (more males than females), women's attitudes toward traditional family sex roles, and being behind grade for age. Both high sex ratio and low male education tend to produce favorable conditions for early marriage, since there are fewer women for available males, and since women tend to enter into unions with men of similar background and educational status (Laumann et al. 1994). These factors also increased Latina females' chances of dropping out of school (Kaplan 1990). Although these variables become important at the macro level of analysis, they are probably not consciously perceived at the micro level, yet they have their effect.

Inclinations toward earlier marriage and childbearing were reflected in the attitudes of African American, Latino, and Asian high school students in Los Angeles who were surveyed about their attitudes toward marriage and childbearing (Erickson 1987). The Latinos and Asians were more similar to each other than to African Americans regarding the age at which they thought females were ready for a sexual relationship. Two-thirds (63%) of Latinos and 82% of Asians thought women should wait until age 18 or older before initiating sexual activity compared to only 30% of African Americans. The Latinos reported younger "ideal" ages for marriage and childbearing than African Americans and Asians. A higher percentage of Latinos (19%) than African Americans (9%) or Asians (10%) thought the ideal age for marriage for a woman was under 21 years of age, although similar proportions of African Americans (17%) and Latinos (17%) thought the ideal age for childbearing was under age 21. Thus, for Latinos, sex, marriage, and childbearing appear to be perceived as coterminous.

As Flores notes:

> Latinas get married at a very early age. The cultural attitude—the sooner the better—is based on the myth that real life starts and culminates with marriage. Worst of all, the Latina does not even imagine that there is anything else but marriage. She goes directly from the domination of her father to the domination of her husband. . . . Marrying young is common, acceptable, encouraged and historically-based. (1990, 47–48)

### Attitudes toward Sexuality

Cultural attitudes toward sexuality are also relevant to adolescent childbearing patterns among Latinas. Several studies suggest that Latinos are conservative in their views on sexual behavior and that the topics of teenage sexual activity and the use of contraceptives by unmarried persons are controversial (Baird 1993; Grebler et al. 1970; Hotvedt 1976; Martinez 1981; Namerow and Philliber 1983). Studies of parent-child communication about sex and birth control suggest that there is very little communication about sex in Latino families (Fennelly 1993). Conservative attitudes toward sex are thought to be stronger among Mexican Americans than other Latino groups (DuRant et al. 1990).

Sexual conservatism is not surprising considering the fact that the dominant religious background of Latinos is Roman Catholicism. The Catholic religion is well known for its conservative views on sex, contraception, and abortion, although many studies suggest that this does not affect fertility patterns, since American Catholics no longer differ from non-Catholics in completed fertility (Alvirez 1973; Amaro 1988; Bean and Tienda 1987; Grebler et al. 1970). Flores (1990) suggests, however, that religion has a strong socialization effect on Latino sexuality and reproductive behavior.

> Growing up Catholic is as much a part of us as growing up Latina. . . . There is a suffocating burden of church-induced guilt among Catholic Latinas. (p. 78)

> . . . we are religiously, culturally and traditionally conditioned to having many children. . . . So for me it was only natural that I would also have many children. More importantly, there was *never* anything said to the contrary. It was always, "You'll have lots of children when you get married." . . . Our belief system said, "Get married and have a big family. God will bless you and you'll be happy." (p. 68)

> Father [the priest] offers one perfect solution [to questions about sex]: Obey, be a dutiful wife and carry out God's will. . . . The one thing the church has vigorously taught is that there shall be no birth control. (p. 83)

Despite the church's teaching on birth control, data on contraceptive use patterns among Latina women suggest that although contraception is rarely used before the first birth, it is completely acceptable for birth spacing or to limit childbearing once the desired family size is reached (Amaro 1988; Erickson and Scrimshaw 1985; Kay 1978; Marin et al. 1981; World Fertility Survey 1980). Although many Latinos are now converting to fundamental Protestant religions, these groups are also quite conservative regarding sexual behavior and gender roles.

Another traditional Latino cultural value is the ideal of "purity" for Latina females. Women are expected to be virgins until they marry. Ideally, young girls are closely watched and chaperoned until marriage. Even after marriage, a young wife is often jealously guarded by her husband until she becomes pregnant and often even longer until she is no longer considered desirable by other men (Bello 1979; Mirande and Enriquez 1979; Pavich 1986; Scrimshaw 1978a). Young women are expected to be modest in their behavior, to know little about sex, and not to enjoy intercourse. The dichotomy between the "good woman" and the "bad woman" is a well known Latino stereotype (Pavich 1986). The good woman is a wife and mother. She is nonerotic, saintly, and virginal. She tolerates her husband's sexual needs and does not develop her own sexuality. She is devoted to her family, and her personal needs are secondary. In contrast, the bad woman is a mistress or a whore. She is erotic and seductive. She enjoys sex and is a willing and responsive sexual partner. In Amaro's (1988) study, Mexican American women in East Los Angeles reported a low level of sexual enjoyment, and most agreed that sex was more a duty than a pleasure, suggesting a continuation of repressive attitudes toward sex for women. Flores summarizes:

> Sex is still referred to by many Latinas as "you-know-what." Latinas are naive about sex. They see it as a duty, thus they don't fake headaches too often. They view sex within marriage as okay because the church says it's okay, but sex before marriage makes them feel guilty. (1990, 60)

Such values may put young Latina women at a disadvantage in the United States, where dating and sexual norms for adolescents are different, and the cultural system of chaperonage (by brothers, aunts, or other family members) cannot be instituted due to constraints of school, work, geographical distance, and the impersonality characterizing urban settings.

### Acceptance of Teenage Motherhood

There is some evidence, from both Mexico and the United States, that despite these conservative views about sexual behavior, once a young unmarried girl becomes pregnant, the family is accepting and supportive after the fact (Felice et al. 1987; Martinez 1981; Moss and Hensleigh 1991; Pavich 1986; Salazar 1979; Smith et al. 1987). Although her sexual behavior might be disapproved and considered shameful, after the initial shock and anger the family eventually supports her and begins to look forward to the birth of the child. Often the girl marries the father of the baby or lives with him in a consensual union. For young girls who are already married, pregnancy is eagerly anticipated, and if it does not occur within the year after marriage, there is great concern about the bride's potential fertility. Culturally, pregnant women are afforded a prestigious position, and great care is taken to assure a healthy birth (see Kay 1978, 1980). For many young women from disadvantaged homes, pregnancy may be the first time in a long time that they have received attention and respect (Speraw 1982). Flores enlightens:

> Latinas assume that being pregnant is one of the greatest things that can happen to them and therefore they should be thankful. Because

of our cultural conditioning, we find ourselves rationalizing: "It's okay to get pregnant without thinking or planning, because that's what I'm supposed to be doing. It is expected and acceptable. I'll be praised for it." . . . [When you are pregnant] *Tú eres una reina* (You are a queen). (1990, 70)

The emerging picture from this review of cultural influences, then, suggests that Latina female teens can be expected to have a strong orientation toward traditional female roles. They tend to enter into marriage, or informal union, and begin their families earlier than what is considered normative for non-Latina whites. Additionally, it appears that earlier school leaving is more acceptable among Latinas and may facilitate earlier family formation, particularly among immigrants.

### Research on Latina
### Adolescent Reproductive Behavior

Although there is a large amount of literature on teenage pregnancy in the United States, most of this research over the past two decades has focused on African American adolescent childbearing and racial differences in reproductive behavior, subsuming Latinas primarily into the white population. As recently as 1986 there was only limited information about Latina adolescent fertility (Darabi et al. 1986). Much has been published since that time, but the literature and research on Latina teenage reproductive behavior lags far behind that on African American teens. This is especially true for studies of adolescent childbearing among Latinas. However, the recent work on Latina teenage pregnancy and sexual behavior, particularly that which addresses acculturation differences, supports the idea that cultural norms and values surrounding reproduction are important factors in Latina teen childbearing.

It is important to note that many analyses of national data until very recently included Latinos of all subgroups, which may mask significant subgroup differences. Since Mexicans are the largest Latino group in the United States (64% of Latinos are of Mexican origin or descent), aggregate data on Latinos tend to reflect the characteristics of this group. Only recently have nationally representative data on Latinos been reported by ethnic subgroup (i.e., Cuban, Mexican, Puerto Rican, and other Latino). Studies of Latinos from distinct geographic areas reflect the predominant group living in that area (e.g., Mexicans in the Midwest and Southwest, Puerto Ricans in the Northeast, Cubans in Miami). These studies have documented differences in reproductive characteristics among Latinos, African

Americans, and non-Latino whites, and considerable variation by Latino subgroup and by acculturation level within these subgroups. The following summary of Latino adolescent reproductive behavior draws on both types of studies.

### Birth Rates

Birth rates to Latina adolescents are high. Among Latinas aged 15 to 19 the birth rate, 100.3 per thousand in 1990, was more similar to the high rate of African Americans, 116.2 per thousand, than to the lower rates of whites, 42.5 per thousand (*MMWR* 1993). Among Latinas, Mexican American adolescents have the highest birth rate (108.0; *MMWR* 1993), and U.S.-born Latina adolescents have almost double the birth rate of the non-U.S.-born (Ventura 1988). Latina and white young women are much more likely to marry during pregnancy than African American women (Fennelly 1993). More births to Latinas are marital births than among other groups (Darabi and Ortiz 1987). Among Mexicans, more than half of births to teens are marital births (Darabi et al. 1986). In California, the rate of illegitimate births for Mexican Americans is the lowest of all ethnic groups: 216.9 per thousand births compared to 335.9 for whites and 555.6 for African Americans (Medina 1979).

### Sexual Behavior

Although birth rates are high, the proportion of sexually active Latina female adolescents is similar to that of whites, and both are much lower than that of African Americans. Nationwide studies have shown that 48% of Latina, and 52% of white, females aged 15–19 have experienced intercourse compared to 61% of African Americans of the same age (Forrest and Singh 1990). Moreover, Latina adolescents have the lowest proportion who were sexually active premaritally, only 30% compared to 55% for African Americans and 36% for whites (Torres and Singh 1986). They also had the highest proportion of teens ever married, 20% compared to 4% for African Americans and 8% for whites (Torres and Singh 1986). Another study, which provided the proportion sexually active by age, noted that at age 15 the proportion sexually active was quite low: 8% for whites, 6% for Latinas, and 13% for African Americans. Among 17-year-old females, 31% of whites, 29% of Latinas, and 46% of African Americans have had sexual intercourse. At age 19, the proportion rose to 66%, 58%, and 79% respectively (Mott and Huarin 1988). Among Latinas, Mexican Americans have the lowest proportion of sexually active female adolescents (DuRant et al. 1990). Among male teens, whites have the lowest proportion sexually active by age 19 (76%),

African Americans the highest (94%), and Latinos intermediate (80%), reflecting the double standard in sexual behavior for male and female Latinos described earlier (Fennelly 1993; Mott and Huarin 1988).

### Contraceptive Use

Several studies have shown that Latina adolescents also have the lowest rates of contraceptive use and tend to initiate contraceptive use a longer time after becoming sexually active than either African American or white teens (Aneshensel et al. 1989; Becerra and de Anda 1984; Namerow and Jones 1982). They are consistently less likely to use birth control at first intercourse (Mosher and Bachrach 1987; Torres and Singh 1986), to use birth control at first premarital intercourse—only 27% compared to 51% of whites and 34% of African Americans (Mosher and McNally 1991)—or to use birth control before having an abortion (Henshaw and Silverman 1988). They are also less likely to go to a family-planning clinic, but if they do, they are more likely to be seeking a pregnancy test than African Americans and whites (Mosher and Horn 1988). Taken together, these factors probably explain the discrepancy between the lower proportions sexually active and the higher birth rates among Latina adolescents.

### Abortion

Data on abortion, especially among adolescents, are difficult to obtain. Henshaw and Silverman (1988) estimated the abortion rate of Latina women of childbearing age at 43 per thousand, higher than the 23 per thousand rate of whites. Studies of small samples of Latina adolescents, however, suggest that they are less likely than whites to use abortion (Aneshensel et al. 1989; Joyce 1988; Leibowitz et al. 1986; Namerow and Jones 1982). Data estimating abortions from the Hispanic Health and Nutrition Examination Study (H-HANES) suggest that among ever-pregnant adolescents, Mexican-origin teens were much less likely than Cubans and Puerto Ricans to have had an abortion (Erickson and Kaplan 1992). Another study of Latina youth in Los Angeles family-planning clinics found that past use of abortion was driven more by gender-role orientation and reproductive variables than by level of acculturation or familism, which is defined as a strong attachment to, emphasis on, and identification with family (Kaplan and Erickson 1997). The higher rate of abortion for Latina women, overall, conflicts with the lower rates reported for Latina adolescents. However, because of cultural attitudes of disapproval regarding abortion, there may be underreporting of abortion by Latina youth. Alternatively, abortion may be used by women to resolve unintended pregnancies later in their childbearing careers. Bearing several children before resorting to birth control or family planning is consistent with cultural values outlined earlier.

## Mexican Americans in the Southwest

Recently, much more research has addressed the Latino adolescent population in the Southwest, coinciding with the rapid growth of the Latino population in this area. These studies parallel the findings of national studies, largely, one might expect, because Latinos of Mexican origin predominate in the Southwest and also constitute the largest proportion of Latinos in the United States (Bean and Tienda 1987). Latina adolescent females in Los Angeles County, for example, have a lower proportion of sexually active individuals than members of other ethnic or racial groups (except Asians) and tend to initiate sexual activity at older ages (Aneshensel et al. 1989; Erickson et al. 1987). Young Latino males, however, show a sexually active proportion similar to that of whites (Erickson et al. 1987). Sexually active Latina females in Los Angeles County are less likely to have used contraception and more likely to have given birth than white females, although they are no more likely to have been pregnant. The difference in fertility was due to the greater use of abortion among non-Latina white teens (Aneshensel et al. 1989).

## Effects of Acculturation

A few studies have begun to address the issue of the variation in sexual behavior between more- and less-acculturated Latinos. In most of these studies, a combination of language preference, country of birth, and length of residence in the United States was used to measure level of acculturation. These studies suggest that the less-acculturated, Spanish-speaking group as a whole is more traditional and conservative in sexual behavior and attitudes toward female roles than the more-acculturated, English-speaking group (DuRant et al. 1990; Rapkin and Erickson 1990). Mexican teens are reported to be the most conservative and traditional of all groups (DuRant et al. 1990; Mott and Mott 1984). A study of family-planning clients (including both adult and adolescent females) found that Spanish-speaking Latina women were more sexually conservative, having fewer lifetime sexual partners and older age at first intercourse than more-acculturated, English-speaking Latinas, who were, in turn, more conservative than non-Latinas (Rapkin and Erickson 1990). Darabi and Ortiz (1987) found that rates of sexual activity increase with generation among Mexican-origin women aged 14 to 22, from 19% for first generation to 41% for third generation, and that the rate of premarital birth was highest among third-generation women. They also found that the bulk of first births to Mexican-origin women were marital births (Darabi and Ortiz 1987). Similarly, in California the proportion of births to Latinas under age 18 is lower among the less acculturated (5.5%) than among the more acculturated (9.3%; Brindis and Jeremy 1988). Another study from Los Angeles suggested that when pregnancy occurs, it is planned to a much greater extent (63%) among Spanish-speaking, less-acculturated Latina adolescents than among either more-acculturated bilingual or English-speaking teens (22%) or among whites (30%; Becerra and de Anda 1984). An Arizona study of primarily in-school Latino youth (i.e., likely to be more acculturated), found that sexual attitudes were governed more by the peer group than by family attitudes (Christopher et al. 1993). Thus, value conflicts may put the more-acculturated Latina teen at increased risk for unintended pregnancy (Darabi and Ortiz 1987; Jacobs 1994). A study of 15-to-24-year-old Latinos in Detroit found that among women, acculturation had a strong positive association with the likelihood of sexual experience (Ford and Norris 1993).

### Birth Outcomes

A few studies have addressed birth outcome among Latina adolescents. They suggest that Latina adolescents share the same pattern of relatively good birth outcomes characteristic of Latina women in general, despite inadequate prenatal care (Erickson 1990; Felice et al. 1986; Williams et al. 1986). The incidence of low birth weight among Latina adolescent births (9.3%) is lower than that among whites (9.8%) or African Americans (14.5%; Balcazar and Aoyama 1991). Low rates among Latina teens are part of the larger paradox of the overall good birth outcomes of Latina women in the United States, despite their higher rates of demographic and perinatal risk factors (Balcazar and Aoyama 1991; Markides and Coreil 1986).

### Summary

Latina female teens living in the United States are less likely to be sexually active than other groups, but once they become sexually active they are less likely to use contraception. If they become pregnant, Latina teens are more likely to carry the pregnancy to term. This results in a high birthrate for Latina adolescents. More of the births to Latinas are marital births than among other groups, however, suggesting the greater involvement of the father of the baby. Pregnancy and marriage are important contributors to the school drop-out rate among Latina females, although dropout is more common before these transitional events. Several studies support the idea that less-acculturated Latinos are more conservative and traditional regarding female roles than the more-acculturated Latinos. Finally, in Latino culture the attitudes toward children and motherhood are reported to be strongly positive, so that the baby's father, his family, and the girl's family tend to be supportive and involved once pregnancy occurs. This pattern is consistent with religious and cultural values about male and female gender roles and the importance of family, marriage, and motherhood that characterize Latino culture.

Thus, teenage pregnancy may be more culturally acceptable within the Latino community, signaling the girl's transition to adulthood rather than being considered a mistake, as it is so often in Anglo middle-class society (Becerra and de Anda 1984; Salazar 1979; Salguero 1984; Scrimshaw 1978b). Finally, there is some evidence that early pregnancy may be consciously chosen and a rational choice within the socioeconomic and cultural context of the lives of Latinos in the United States. Whether planned or unplanned, within marriage or without, pregnancy usually signals a young Latina's transition from childhood to adulthood and ends her formal education.

## CHAPTER THREE

# The East Los Angeles Repeat-Pregnancy Prevention Project

In 1985 there were about three thousand births to women aged 19 and under at Women's Hospital in East Los Angeles, of which about one thousand were to teens aged 17 and under. Pat Jamieson, the health educator at the hospital's family planning clinic, decided that a special repeat-pregnancy prevention program was needed for teens giving birth at the hospital because she was concerned about two groups that, it seemed to her, were becoming increasingly common on the postpartum ward: (1) teens who already had one or more children and (2) teens under the age of 15.

At that time, Women's Hospital[1] was probably the largest delivery hospital in the United States, averaging about sixteen thousand deliveries a year and accounting for about 17% of births in Los Angeles County (LAC). It was a public hospital, part of the L.A. County health system,[2] and was one of the teaching hospitals for the University of Southern California (USC) Medical and Nursing Schools. As part of the larger LAC-USC Medical Center, Women's Hospital provided obstetric and gynecological care and had a family planning clinic on site.[3] Since it was a teaching hospital, research and training were primary activities. Women's Hospital was also the major referral hospital within the county health system for women of high medical risk. Thus, the hospital served not only the poorest of the poor but also the sickest of the sick, and provided them with the latest and best in medical care.

The population of women using the hospital included immigrants primarily from Mexico and Central America, Latinas born in the United States, and a small proportion of African American and other groups. The immigrant population included both documented and undocumented women, although patients/clients were never asked for proof of citizenship.[4] The documented are those who reside in the United States legally. Many have lived uthern California for a number of years and are either already citizens the process of legalization through the Immigration Reform and Con- Act (IRCA) of 1986. The undocumented population does not reside legally in the United States. They crossed the border undetected (designated EWI, "entered without inspection," by the Immigration and Naturalization Service), or they entered with a visa but stayed after its expiration. The undocumented include those who are more recently arrived, those who do not qualify for amnesty under IRCA, and those who do not qualify for political asylum. The undocumented group is an extremely disadvantaged group because of its "underground" status. Ever-tighter restrictions and larger fines for hiring illegal aliens instituted during the late 1980s made it increasingly difficult for them to find work in the Los Angeles area. After the 1994 passage of Proposition 187, which sought to deny health, educational, and social services to illegal residents, hostility toward illegal immigrants, particularly Latinos, heightened considerably. Patients must now prove eligibility for all but emergency services.

The legal residents and citizens served by the hospital are also a disadvantaged group. Los Angeles has a large working-class and middle-class Latino population who are separated economically (through access to private health care) and geographically (through residential neighborhood) from the group served by the hospital. The Latino population served by the family planning clinic at Women's Hospital tends to be extremely disadvantaged economically. They are primarily the working poor without health insurance and the Medicaid-eligible. Most reside in the ghetto areas and housing projects closest to the hospital. Thus, they are plagued by the poverty, drugs, gangs, and violence so commonly found in American inner-city areas.

The young mothers in our project were recruited on the labor and delivery wards at Women's Hospital after they gave birth. They are representative of the population of women described above. Some are only recently arrived and speak only Spanish. Others were born here or have lived here since they were small children and are bilingual. A few speak only English. Some are from the war-ravaged countries of Central America; others have migrated from Mexico in search of a better life. Some are married; some live with their baby's father; others live with their own family. Some were in school when they became pregnant, but most were not. What they have in common is poverty and the fact that they became mothers before their eighteenth birthday.

### Repeat-Pregnancy Prevention in a Clinic Setting

In this section I describe the evolution of our intervention efforts with Latina teen mothers in the family planning clinic. Since no internal funding was available for special services for teen mothers, funds had to be solicited from outside sources—primarily private foundations—that were interested in adolescent childbearing issues. Most foundations provide support for demonstration projects for only limited time periods (usually one or two years). If the resulting project cannot be absorbed by the recipient institution when funding ends, which is most often the case, other sources of funding must be sought. For this reason, there were three different intervention projects between 1986 and 1991, each of which was funded by a different foundation and each of which had slightly different goals. Although we referred to them collectively as the "Teen Project," each specific project had its own label, which most often was the name of the funder. In addition, I had a small research project in 1992 that was not aimed at intervention. Each of these four projects resulted in the data on which this book is based, and each is described below.

I became involved with the family planning clinic as a consultant. I was still in graduate school at UCLA at the time, and my doctoral studies in public health focused on Latino reproductive health and teenage pregnancy. The first grant proposal I wrote was submitted to the Los Angeles Regional Family Planning Council, Inc. (LARFPC) for a small amount of funding for the first teenage-pregnancy prevention project at the hospital.

### The LARFPC Project, 1986–1987

The family planning clinic at Women's Hospital had long had a postpartum ward outreach program in which all women delivering at the hospital—which then averaged between fifty and sixty deliveries a day—were visited in the hospital and given foam and condoms, instruction on how and why to use them, and an appointment for postpartum care. Most women were given appointments at the clinics in which they received prenatal care throughout Los Angeles County.[5] Those who were medically high-risk, those who had had cesarean sections, and those who had received no prenatal care were given appointments at the family planning clinic at Women's Hospital.

We piggybacked our LARFPC teen project onto the ward outreach program to provide intensified services to teen mothers aged 17 and under and to provide contraceptive case management to teens who returned to our clinic for postpartum care. Two primary goals were to encourage return for the postpartum appointment and to facilitate contraceptive use in order to prevent a repeat pregnancy for a minimum of two years. A secondary goal was to promote school return, job skills, and English skills to facilitate self-sufficiency.

The LARFPC project had two bilingual family planning counselors, called "teen outreach workers" (TOWs), who were specially trained to work with teens. They visited each teen aged 17 and under on the postpartum ward and involved her in what was by hospital standards a lengthy (30–45-minute) interview. The interview covered her current social situation, reproductive history and plans, contraceptive history and plans, and her plans for school, employment, and the future. Next, the TOWs provided information about contraceptive methods and gave the teen a supply of foam and condoms for use if she had sex before she came to her postpartum appointment. Finally, the teen received a postpartum appointment at the appropriate clinic. The counselors took a Polaroid picture of each teen with her infant (if in the room) and placed the picture, along with the place, time, and date of the postpartum appointment and the counselor's name and phone number, in a folder that was given to the young woman.

Two weeks prior to the postpartum appointment each teen who had an appointment at Women's Hospital for postpartum care was called at home to remind her of the time and day of her appointment and to offer assistance with any problems she might have. At the postpartum appointment a TOW counseled the client regarding birth control and became her contraceptive case manager and contact person in the clinic. The TOW would see her client each time she came to the clinic and would refer her for special needs that could not be met in-clinic. The TOWs were given the time and flexibility to address the needs of the teen clients. For example, they were able to spend thirty to sixty minutes with each client if needed and to see teens who came without an appointment. In this way we hoped to remove service barriers to contraceptive care and to help teens prevent repeat pregnancies.

In 1986–1987, the TOWs interviewed over 1,017 teens on the postpartum ward, representing about 90% of the deliveries to teens under age 18. The ward outreach and telephone follow-up increased the teen postpartum return rate at the family planning clinic from under 50% to 64%. However, just increasing compliance with the postpartum visit, while a necessary intermediate variable, was far less than what, over time, we realized was necessary for consistent, effective contraceptive use among this population. In fact, we found that we needed to address a myriad of social and economic problems before the teens could focus on contraception. In order to effect contraceptive use we were forced to respond to their social and economic needs. This led to the expansion of the LARFPC Project to include high-risk case management. The TOWs were absorbed by the family planning clinic.

### High-Risk Case Management, 1987–1988

In 1987 the Teen Project was expanded with funding from the Joseph Drown Foundation and the California Community Foundation to include a high-risk case manager for sixty-five of the highest-risk teen mothers. High-risk criteria included any one or more of the following: (1) less than 16 years old, (2) multiparous teen (more than one child) or teen with multiple birth (e.g., twins), (3) serious medical problems of teen (e.g., diabetes, leukemia), (4) serious medical problems of infant (e.g., prematurity, low birth weight), (5) inadequate social support system, (6) extreme poverty, (7) substance abuse, (8) suicidal ideation, (9) sexual abuse, (10) physical abuse, and (11) subsequent pregnancy.

The high-risk manager was a bilingual, bicultural male with a master's degree in social psychology and experience in health education, social service referral, and follow-up. He networked with existing agencies and service providers to link clients with the resources they required. Case management began with a needs assessment and the development of an individual case plan. The case manager and the client worked as a team in negotiating the health, educational, and social service system. The case manager maintained, minimally, bimonthly contact with each client, found appropriate referrals for identified problems, integrated the teen into appropriate agencies, and motivated her to use the services available. Through the more intimate relationship that developed between the case manager and the high-risk teens, we were introduced to the sad fact that many (about one-third) of the high-risk teens had been sexually and/or physically abused. Funding for this program ended in 1990, and the cost could not be absorbed by the clinic. This was unfortunate because the program showed success, especially in promoting school return (Erickson and Reyes 1990). We were fortunate, however, to have the services of a hospital social worker one day a week who continued to provide crisis care. In the beginning of 1988, internal funding pressures insured that outside funding would be required to continue providing special services to teen mothers, and I wrote a proposal that was funded by The William and Flora Hewlett Foundation.

### The Hewlett Project, 1989–1991

In December 1988 we received a three-year grant from The William and Flora Hewlett Foundation to evaluate the effectiveness of the overall program in preventing repeat pregnancies. The Hewlett grant provided support for four TOWs and the research staff. I was a co-investigator on this project and was responsible for research, evaluation, and overall project coordination.[6] The project was designed as a clinical intervention program with the major focus on the collection of quantitative data for evaluation purposes. As the project proceeded, however, I began more and more to use the qualitative research methods in which I had also been trained, because the program, as designed, did not seem to fit the needs of the young women it served, and because the quantitative data were not explaining what I considered some of the more interesting questions about the relationship of cultural norms and values to the experience of these young mothers.

The Hewlett Project used a quasi-random method for assigning teens aged 17 and under recruited on the postpartum ward to either a case or control group. Every third teen interviewed became part of the control group unless she was determined to be high-risk. All high-risk teens were assigned to the case group. New mothers who received appointments to the hospital clinic were interviewed on the postpartum ward within twenty-four hours of giving birth and again at follow-up family planning visits thereafter. While all teens were interviewed on the postpartum ward, only the cases received the intensive follow-up. After the initial interview, the controls were given regular care in the family planning clinic. The primary difference in care between the case and control groups was that the cases received intensive personalized follow-up at regular intervals. They were also called if an appointment were broken, and they received referrals to outside agencies for special needs (e.g., food, housing, Medi-Cal [California's Medicaid program], school, child care, etc.). In regular care, follow-up was only provided for medical reasons.

The protocol for the Hewlett Project included the postpartum outreach described earlier, the postpartum visit, and additional contacts made following the postpartum family planning visit at regular, designated intervals (see Table 3.1). In addition, the TOWs had a maximum caseload of sixty teens to allow them the considerable amount of time required by the follow-up protocols. The Hewlett Project ended in December of 1991 and served 485 teens over its three years of operation, 308 cases and 177 controls (see Table 3.2).[7]

## Systematic Data Collection, 1992

In the summer of 1992, I returned to Los Angeles to do a follow-up, exploratory study probing more deeply into the cultural meanings attached to contraceptive methods, women's roles, and life-event norms. The study used systematic data collection techniques, which are designed to explore the cognitive patterns underlying the domain under study (see Weller and Romney 1988).[8] Twenty-eight teen clients and thirteen family planning providers participated in the study.

## Methods and Procedures

This section describes the methods and procedures used in data collection and analysis.

Table 3.1.    Summary of Intervention Schedule for the 1989–1991 Hewlett Project

| Time of Contact | Type of Contact | Case | Control |
|---|---|---|---|
| | *First Year of Project* | | |
| Delivery | Personal Chart Review | TOW[†] | TOW |
| 2 weeks PP* | Telephone | TOW | TOW |
| 3 weeks PP | Telephone | TOW | |
| PP Visit | Personal | TOW | |
| 6 weeks PP | Telephone | TOW | |
| 8 weeks PP | Telephone | TOW | |
| Variable per medical protocol | Personal/Telephone | TOW | |
| 3, 6, 9 months PP | Telephone | TOW | |
| 12 months PP | Telephone | TOW | TOW |
| | *Second Year of Project* | | |
| Variable per medical protocol | Personal/Telephone | TOW | |
| 15, 18, 21 months PP | Telephone | TOW | |
| 24 months PP | Telephone | TOW | TOW |
| | *Third Year of Project* | | |
| Variable per medical protocol | Personal/Telephone | TOW | |
| 27, 30, 33 months PP | Telephone | TOW | |
| 36 months PP | Telephone | TOW | TOW |

*PP = postpartum
[†]TOW = teen outreach worker

Table 3.2.    Hewlett Project Recruitment, 1989–1991

| Recruitment Period | Cases | Controls | Total |
|---|---|---|---|
| 4/89–12/89 | 114 | 66 | 180 |
| 1/90–12/90 | 132 | 74 | 206 |
| 1/91–6/91 | 62 | 37 | 99 |
| Total | 308 | 177 | 485 |

## The Postpartum Ward Surveys, 1986–1987 and 1992–1994

A total of 1,017 Latina teens aged 17 and under were interviewed during their postpartum hospital stay between October 1986 and December 1987 as part of the LARFPC Project, and another 1,293 between January 1992 and November 1994 as part of the second Hewlett Project. This represents 90% of the teens who delivered at the hospital during those time periods. Those who were not interviewed were missed either due to staff illness or quick

Table 3.3.     Data-Collection Methods and Procedures, Hewlett Project, 1989–1991

| Quantitative | Qualitative |
|---|---|
| **Method** | |
| Surveys (TOWs*) | Informal Reviews (TOWs, I‡) |
| Medical record review (RAs†) | Key informant interview (I) |
| | Participant observation (I) |
| | Direct observation (I) |
| **Type of Data** | |
| Computer Data Files (RAs) | Written field notes (I) |
| | Longitudinal case files (TOWs) |

*TOWs = teen outreach workers
†RAs = research assistants
‡I = investigator (author)

turnaround between delivery and discharge, which was sometimes as little as twelve hours.

The survey was implemented by bilingual, bicultural family planning workers and collected a set of standardized information on demographic variables, prenatal care, birth outcome, the teen mother's relationship to the baby's father and to her family of origin, reproductive and contraceptive history and plans, and school status. Information on birth outcome was abstracted from the medical record.

The survey data were analyzed using the Statistical Analysis System (SAS), a widely used statistical package available for both mainframe and personal computers. Analysis included descriptive statistics (e.g., frequency distributions, means).

### The Hewlett Project, 1989–1991

Table 3.3 provides a summary of the variety of quantitative and qualitative research methods that were used in data collection and indicates which member of the research team was responsible for collecting the data. Each of these methods is described below.

#### Surveys

The surveys included the postpartum ward survey used in the 1986–1987 study described above and six follow-up instruments for use at different periods during the study. The surveys were implemented by the bilingual, bicultural family planning counselors (TOWs) at each contact with the teen. The surveys summarized a set of standardized information on each teen at each contact as shown in the following outline:

Informal Interview Format, Hewlett Project, 1989–1991

I.  Introduction

TOW introduces herself and establishes rapport with client.

II.  Topics to Be Covered
   A.  Child's health
   B.  Mother's health
   C.  Problems/needs TOW can address
   D.  Relationship to father of baby/significant other
   E.  Relationship to family
   F.  Living arrangements
   G.  Birth control and sexual activity
   H.  Pregnancy status
   I.  Work and/or education
   J.  Breast-feeding (when appropriate)

III.  *Adiós*
   A.  Reinforce TOW as contact person in medical system
   B.  Request change of address or telephone number
   C.  Remind teen of next appointment date and inquire about transportation difficulties
   D.  Make referrals (if needed)

Thus, a longitudinal database was built for each case. (Appendix I provides a list of the different survey tools, the follow-up period at which they were implemented, and a summary of major variables.) Data from these surveys were coded and entered into a computer database by a research assistant.

In addition to these more formal surveys, the TOWs often informally interviewed the young women and wrote notes in their project record. Each teen designated as a case had a project record that contained all of the surveys completed with her. This record was kept separate from the medical record because it contained a wide variety of information not relevant for clinical care. Because it was not a medical record, it was available only to the research staff, thus providing a measure of confidentiality.

*Medical Record Review*

Medical records were used in two ways. At the initial interview on the postpartum ward, the TOW abstracted information about the pregnancy, labor and delivery, and baby's condition. The family planning clinic medical record was also reviewed at twelve and twenty-four months postpartum to abstract information about pregnancy tests, diagnosis of repeat pregnancy, diagnosis of sexually transmitted diseases, contraceptive method(s) dispensed, and number of client visits. These medical record abstractions were the only data collected on the control subjects after their initial interview aside from the one- and two-year follow-up telephone calls. The data were entered into a computer database and were used in conjunction with the project record to evaluate the success of the Teen Project in preventing repeat pregnancy. Medical record abstraction was performed by masters-level students from the UCLA School of Public Health.

### Informal Interviews

Much informal interviewing took place at different levels within the project. As noted, the TOWs often interviewed the young women informally, following up on interests of their own. They kept case summaries of their particular caseload. Because they developed a relationship with these young women over time, the TOWs could provide a wealth of information about the more qualitative aspects of these girls' lives. Similarly, I often informally interviewed the staff regarding the program and specific teens within the program to follow up on information that was interesting or important but not necessarily covered in the survey data. While I occasionally talked with individual teens, the majority of direct work with the teens was done by the TOWs in their role as family planning care providers, and they were my key informants.

### Participant and Direct Observation

Because of the building layout and constraints of space in the clinic, the entire Teen Project was housed in one room along with the computer. I worked in this room about once a week. This provided a wonderful opportunity for observing the interactions between the TOWs and the teens and for some firsthand involvement with the young mothers.

In sum, the data are both quantitative and qualitative. In most cases the qualitative data gathering was directed toward making sense of the quantitative data. As both anthropologist and public health professional, I had two different agenda in carrying out this research. First, I became involved in the research as a public health professional, and I wanted to demonstrate the efficacy of the intervention program through conventional quasi-experimental design and quantitative evaluation. This focused the data collection on measurable outcomes such as clinic return, number of visits, and repeat pregnancy.

While analysis of these quantitative data was sufficient for traditional evaluation procedures and for making a contribution to the field of teen pregnancy prevention, I also added a considerable number of sociodemographic variables, such as social support and feelings about pregnancy, that contributed immensely to the richness of the data. These variables addressed my second agenda, understanding the context of teen pregnancy, but they were much more than what was necessary for the program evaluation.

In fact, the magnitude of data collection became burdensome on the staff, who considered their primary loyalties to be to the clients rather than to the research. My anthropological side wanted to be able to understand the quantitative findings better and interpret them in a more meaningful way, and even the additional sociodemographic variables in the interviews were not enough to make sense of what we were finding. Thus, as seemingly paradoxical findings came up, I began asking the TOWs questions aimed at understanding the motivations behind the behavioral outcomes that constituted the quantitative data. As the study progressed and the TOWs began to understand the kind of information I was looking for, they became increasingly adept at analyzing their own and the teens' culture. Two of them had themselves been teenage mothers, and they could translate the experience of teenage pregnancy for me. The coordinating TOW, in particular, provided many insights on the cultural pressures involved in sex and reproduction among Latinos.

*Data Analysis*

The quantitative survey data were analyzed using the Statistical Analysis System (SAS). Analysis included descriptive statistics, chi-square measures of association for nominal data, Student's *t* tests, and ANOVA (Analysis of Variance) tests of the difference between means to explore differences between more- and less-acculturated teens on continuous variables (age, birth weight). Multivariate regression and logistic regression were used to understand the contribution of different variables to outcome measures (the relative contribution of age, acculturation, social support, etc., to adequacy of prenatal care).

The major thrust of the quantitative analysis is a comparison between the Spanish-speaking, more recent immigrants and the bilingual or English-speaking, more-acculturated teens who have lived in the United States since at least 12 years of age.

Qualitative data were analyzed through content analysis of interviews, chart notes, and field notes.

### Systematic Data Collection, 1992

In July and August of 1992, twenty-eight teens and thirteen family planning providers participated in the study. The teens were recruited from among the clients attending the Teen Clinic at Women's Hospital in Los Angeles for family planning care. The providers were on staff at the clinic (nurses, community health workers, health educators). Respondents were asked about three domains of interest: contraceptive methods, women's roles, and life events. First they sorted items in the domain with respect to their similarity (free sort). Then they were asked to rank-order contraceptive methods by efficacy, safety, and use preference; women's roles by importance; and life events by the order in which they should and actually did occur. The names of the items were typed on small cards in English and Spanish, and the participants physically sorted and ordered the items. During the exercises, respondents were interviewed about their reasons for sorting and ranking items as they did, and comments made while performing the tasks were documented. These systematic data were collected by the author and were analyzed using ANTHROPAC—a software program designed specifically to handle this type of data (Borgatti 1992)—using PC SAS, and through content analysis of field notes.

## Protection of Human Subjects

All participants in these studies took part voluntarily. There were no refusals to participate. Project case files and computer identification numbers were securely locked in the project office. Records in the computerized data file were identified by a number not related to the client's medical identification number or any other personal identifying number. Only the researchers and Teen Project staff had access to the files. Medical records of family planning clients were kept with the clinic's patient files in locked cabinets.

The results of these studies are presented using both quantitative and qualitative data to describe and explain the findings. Case studies and the comments and interpretations of the TOWs and other clinic personnel are used throughout as examples illustrating different points. All names, except those of the research staff, are fictitious. Many of the details presented in the case histories have been changed to protect participant confidentiality.

## CHAPTER FOUR

# Los Angeles, the Hospital, and the Research Team

## Los Angeles

Los Angeles, the City of the Angels, better known as "L.A." to its residents, is the second largest city in the United States. The metropolitan area is huge, covering 4,070 square miles, and the freeway system legendary. The county of Los Angeles, which is roughly coterminous with the larger metropolitan area, has a population of almost nine million, 40% of which is Latino. Thus, Los Angeles has been called the "Chicano capital of the United States" (Moore and Vigil 1993).

But it is also a "global city" (Moore and Pinderhughes 1993), made up of a multitude of smaller cities, each with its own distinct character. Some, like Hollywood, Beverly Hills, Watts, and Venice Beach, are familiar to most Americans. Others are residential areas that are less familiar—West L.A. between Santa Monica and Beverly Hills, where UCLA is located; the San Fernando Valley, a large valley on the other side of the coastal mountains and Hollywood Hills; Silver Lake in the downtown hill area near Griffith Park. Still others are ethnic or racial enclaves, such as Chinatown (downtown near the government buildings); Koreatown (between downtown and the Miracle Mile area); Little Tokyo (downtown near the train station); East L.A. (on the east side of the L.A. River that divides the downtown area, and near LAC-USC Medical Center) and adjacent Montebello, which are primarily Mexican Latino; little El Salvador (between the Harbor Freeway and Koreatown); and Westwood Boulevard in West L.A. near UCLA, which has a significant Middle Eastern, especially Iranian, presence. These are characterized primarily by a core of ethnically oriented and owned businesses surrounded by a residential section. As in most large cities, these neighborhoods are constantly changing as the demographic picture of the city changes. For example, South Central L.A., which was primarily African American in the

1960s, has now become about half African American and half Latino. The ebb and flow of different cultural and ethnic groups in different geographic areas creates tension and conflict, creativity and collaboration. It is an exciting place in which to experience the processes of culture contact, acculturation, biculturalism, and assimilation.

East L.A., 94% Latino by 1980, and the adjacent central city area were heavily settled by immigrants from Mexico and Central America in the 1970s and 1980s (Chinchilla et al. 1993; Moore and Vigil 1993). The majority of immigrants were from Mexico, and this "Mexicanization" of the central city area has had an economic and cultural impact. The area is very poor, and culturally it is traditionally Mexican. The farther east one goes from this central area, the less immigrant dominated and poverty stricken the Latino neighborhoods become (Moore and Vigil 1993).

The Latino sections capture the flavor of Latin American cities. Little El Salvador, near MacArthur Park, is Central American in character, with its *botánicas* (herbal stores), *espiritistas* (spiritists), salsa music, and *pupusas* (a Salvadoran specialty food). East L.A., near Women's Hospital, is primarily Mexican and Mexican American and has its own special cultural feel, which Cheech Marin portrayed well in the popular film *Born in East L.A.* The Mexican American *cholo(a)* style (tattoos, low-rider cars, typical dress style, including white T-shirts and baggy black pants worn low for males and tight jeans, spandex, and big earrings for females) intersperses with more traditional Mexican styles of dress. Older, immigrant women wear *rebozos* (shawls, often covering the head) and a particular style of earrings (long gold earrings set with colorful stones) popular in Mexico. Many of the men wear cowboy boots, hats, and western-style shirts, a style of dress common to northern Mexico. Mariachi bands and strolling guitarists play in the public parks. Mexican food, from the tacos sold by street vendors to the *haute cuisine* of Tamayo's (an upscale restaurant in East L.A.), is available everywhere.

The Catholic parishes are an important and vital part of social life in the Latino areas of L.A. These Latino sections of the city seem much more alive than other areas. People of all ages can be seen out on the streets walking, talking, and shopping. Children are everywhere—running, playing, running errands, baby-sitting the smaller ones. Street vendors sell *palitas* (Popsicles) in exotic flavors like mango, tamarind, and coconut. Others sell fresh fruit, with or without chile and salt, or *refrescos* like lemonade, *jamaica* (hibiscus flavored), and *orchata* (rice water flavored with cinnamon and sugar). It is quite like being in Latin America. Indeed, L.A. has the largest Mexican and largest Salvadoran population outside the borders of those two countries.

It would be difficult for anyone to live in Los Angeles without being influenced at least in some way by Latino culture, and in particular by Mexican culture. California, after all, was once part of Mexico, and the earliest non–Native American settlers were Jesuit priests from Spain and ranchers from Mexico. It was not until the gold rush that large numbers of Anglos entered the state for the first time. Mexican influence in cooking, place names, language, architecture, and art is readily apparent. There is a constant flow back and forth across the border with Mexico, further enriching and renewing Latino culture in L.A. Spanish radio and television stations are numerous. There are bilingual personnel in practically all businesses, hospitals, and government institutions. It is often said that a Spanish speaker could spend his or her whole life in L.A. never having to learn English. This has both advantages and disadvantages, however, because English is still the key to full participation in American society.

The Latino population is a young population with higher fertility than Anglos, and Latino children outnumber all others in public schools, constituting 70% of the city school population in 1991 (Moore and Vigil 1993). The emerging Latino professional class is becoming more apparent, and much more social mixing among racial and ethnic groups occurs in this class than among the lower and middle classes. Middle- and upper-class households of all racial and ethnic compositions have come to rely on Latina women as maids and baby-sitters, and Latino males provide much of the manual labor in the city. They are gardeners, restaurant workers, parking attendants, construction workers, janitors, and casual laborers. Wave after wave of new immigrants comes to L.A. from Mexico and Central America, providing a constant pool of cheap labor for domestic services, day labor, and agricultural work. With each new wave, cultural traditions are renewed and the Spanish language revitalized. Even when young, upwardly mobile Latinos move away from the barrios to middle-class areas, they leave behind family, friends, and the Catholic parishes to which they retain close ties (Moore and Vigil 1993). Bilingualism and biculturalism are the hallmarks of the emerging Latino middle class, not assimilation to Anglo culture.

I lived in Los Angeles for thirteen years, between 1978 and 1991 (1978–1984 in Venice and 1984–1991 in West L.A.). During that time, I witnessed the huge influx of immigrants from Mexico, Central America, the Middle East, and Asia, and the widening gap between the rich and the poor. As more Latino immigrants came in, African Americans were displaced both numerically in terms of the proportion of the population and physically in neighborhoods, steadily losing ground to the new immigrants. Latinos are now the largest minority population in Los Angeles, and for the first time since California was part of Mexico, the proportion of whites is less than the combined proportion of minorities. Thus, L.A. is truly a multicultural city, and underlying this multicultural reality is an uneasy tension among the different groups. Poverty, disenfranchisement, and tension erupted into violence, arson, and looting in May 1992 in response to the Rodney King verdict[1] in South Central L.A., the same area where the Watts riots of the 1960s took place. These two riots have been called the worst urban riots in the history of the United States.

Increasing violence and hostility toward Latinos has emerged since the 1994 passage of Proposition 187, which sought to deny health, educational, and social services to illegal residents. Many Anglos, now in the minority, are afraid of the loss of their own culture and position. Much of the debate over English is an attempt to legislate the cultural dominance of Anglo America, for language is culture. Many others welcome Latinos and the multicultural city that L.A. is becoming (Hurtado et al. 1992).

The economic decline in L.A. is part of the overall recession experienced by the whole country since the late 1980s, but it came a bit later to California (the early 1990s). State, county, and municipal budgets are being cut back. The gap between the rich and the poor is widening. California has steadily lost its industrial base as business and industry moved to areas with cheaper labor and cheaper real estate. In the 1980s the real estate market was so inflated that it was nearly impossible for most families in California to purchase a home, and rents were very high, forcing families, relatives, and friends to live together in overcrowded conditions. As the industrial base moved out, fewer people could find well-paying jobs. The health care crisis is acute in L.A., with public hospitals all but bankrupt. More than 2.5 million Angelenos are uninsured, most of them workers and their dependents.[2] The poor slipped deeper into poverty, and the rich became ever richer during the 1980–1988 Reagan administration and the 1988–1992 Bush administration. The disparity of wealth in L.A. is obscene, and it is no surprise to anyone even remotely aware of how economically desperate millions of residents are that the massive looting (primarily of such necessities as food, clothing, and household appliances) occurred during the 1992 riots. Exacerbating this, especially after the Immigration Reform and Control Act (IRCA),[3] is the increasing population of illegal residents who form an "underground" population unable to work legally in the United States, without hope of becoming citizens and without resources to survive. There is debate about whether or not the increasing crackdown on illegals has made any impact on illegal immigration.

### The Hospital Setting

The LAC-USC Family Planning Clinic is a Title X–funded public clinic located in Women's Hospital on Mission and Zonal in East L.A.[4] The hospital is part of the larger LAC-USC Medical Center, which includes a general hospital, a pediatric hospital, a psychiatric hospital, medical and nursing schools, and a variety of out-patient clinics. The family planning clinic is situated on the ground floor near the emergency room. The obstetrics and gynecology clinic is located across the main hall from the family planning clinic. Labor and delivery is located on the fourth floor, and postpartum patients recover on the fourth and fifth floors. The Medical Center serves a primarily Latino population (80% to 90%), which is predominantly of Mexican origin or descent.

During the day there are always large numbers of patients, their partners or friends who accompany them to the clinic, and small children in the halls and waiting areas. Pregnant women can be seen waiting for appointments, sitting in groups talking to other women, or knitting baby things. Women in the early stages of labor appear anxious as they wait to be admitted or walk the halls to facilitate the progress of labor. Throughout the day attendants push pregnant women in wheelchairs into the hospital and wheel women and their newborns who have been discharged from the hospital outside where family and friends await them. Volunteers circulate with magazines and flowers; technicians hurry to the lab with blood samples; and housekeeping is constantly cleaning and performing routine maintenance in this overburdened facility.

It is important to convey the Latino flavor of the setting. By way of illustration, on one evening, I remember leaving the clinic quite late (sometime after 9:00 P.M.) after spending hours immersed in a logic problem with the database system. I walked from the quiet, deserted clinic into the hospital waiting room and became momentarily disoriented. Everyone appeared to be Mexican, and Spanish was the only language being spoken. I had also been doing some consulting work on a teen project in Mexico City and was unsure for several painful moments whether I was in Mexico or in Los Angeles. An English announcement on the hospital paging system reoriented me, but that incident stands out in my mind as one of the best examples of the extent to which many parts of L.A. are thoroughly Latino.

Hospital personnel are easily identified by the badge that each is required to wear. These identification badges display the person's name, job title, and a photograph. Even without the badges, however, it is easy to distinguish the staff by their race, manner of dress, and use of English. Aside from the obvious hospital uniforms (surgical greens, stethoscopes, white coats), the staff dress in a different style than the patients. Men wear suits and ties, and women wear dresses, suits, and other appropriate business attire of significantly better quality and more up-to-date style than that of the low-income patients. Staff converse in English, patients primarily in Spanish. Staff are also more racially heterogeneous than are patients and include a rainbow coalition of Caucasians, African Americans, Latinos, Asians, and Pacific Islanders from the United States and abroad.

The family planning clinic waiting room is an extension of a long hall off the main entrance hallway. Since the clinic is so near the emergency room, the hall must always be kept clear in case of emergency. This is a source of constant problems requiring staff vigilance to keep patients, but especially children, from blocking the hall, although the recent addition of a day care center for patients' children has considerably alleviated this situation. At the end of the hall is the reception desk with a counter and a wall of glass that separates the three receptionists from clients. Patients must speak through holes in the glass, and it is often quite difficult to hear the receptionists on the other side.

On any given day about half of the clients sitting in the forty to fifty chairs lining the hallway are women, some breast-feeding newborns, who are waiting to be seen for their postpartum appointments. The rest are continuing contraceptive clients in various stages of their reproductive careers. Most are accompanied by young children not yet in school. It is very rare to see a teen client in the clinic who is not either a teen mother or a post-SAB follow-up (medical check after a spontaneous abortion). In the ten years I have been involved with the clinic there have been only a handful of teen clients who had come to the clinic for contraception before they became pregnant, and most of these had had a pregnancy "scare." Primary prevention clients—those who had never had a baby and were there for prevention—were a matter for serious celebration among the staff.

Among patients, Spanish is the primary language, although many also speak English, particularly among the teens. Health care providers usually converse among themselves in English, but most are able to speak Spanish as well. Their Spanish ability ranges from bilingual to "able to provide instructions while conducting a physical exam," but they all try. Reflecting the class structure of the dominant society, all the physicians who have regular roles in the clinic are white.[5] The medical director is a white male who speaks only a few words of Spanish. The primary physician in the clinic is a white female who is fluent in Spanish. The nursing staff is more heterogeneous, including one white, one Korean, and two Mexican American nurse practitioners. All are female and speak Spanish. Nearly all of the community workers, family planning counselors, and receptionists are bilingual and bicultural. Most are Mexican American. The bilingual clinic administrator, a registered nurse with a master's degree in public health, is of Cuban origin although born in the United States.

In the clinic waiting area the VCR (videocassette recorder) is constantly playing health education videos in Spanish about reproduction, contraception, sexually transmitted diseases, and AIDS. Babies cry, children shuffle about, and the sounds of ringing telephones and the hospital paging system are ever present. As in most public hospitals, furnishings are functional but drab.

The clinic is open from 8:00 A.M. to 5:00 P.M. daily and uses an appointment system. Specialty clinics such as the diabetic clinic and postpartum clinic are held on specific days. Since the Medical Center is the major teaching hospital for USC, and many of the faculty are leading medical researchers, research projects and clinical trials of contraceptive methods, drugs, and clinical procedures are frequently in progress. For example, Women's Hospital was one of the U.S. sites for clinical trials of RU486 and NORPLANT.[6] It also serves as a county training site for practitioners who want to learn the surgical techniques necessary for inserting and removing the implants. More recently, the clinic was involved with a clinical trial testing the efficacy of antibiotic prophylaxis during IUD (intrauterine device) insertions.

Thus, since both staff and patients were accustomed to the research priorities of the institution and many had participated in them, it was not unusual to undertake a special teen pregnancy prevention project in the clinic setting. Four counselors (the TOWs) were hired exclusively for the Teen Project. They were provided with their own room in an area separate from the regular clinic in which to see the teen clients assigned to the case group. The TOWs are housed in a long, narrow, windowless room with five desks facing the wall, separated from each other by partitions for counseling purposes, although it is still possible to overhear consultations in the next cubicle. A computer for project use is also found in this room. The furniture in the teen room was bought for the Teen Project and is somewhat nicer than other clinic furnishings. The desks are off-white with locking shelves overhead and locking drawers to the right. Each desk has a telephone equipped with the six clinic lines, although often all the lines are in use. Chairs and divider partitions are upholstered in a pleasant mauve color. Several locking, industrial gray file cabinets hold the case records. Posters on the walls convey family planning, breast-feeding, and STI (sexually transmitted infection) messages. Each TOW has added her own decorations, including pictures of family and friends, pictures of important events (weddings, graduations), and other items of personal interest. The room is referred to by staff as the "Teens." In contrast, the regular clinic has one large counseling room with about twenty desks separated by partitions forming cubicles. This room also houses the photocopy machine and a computer that is part of the on-line hospital network system. It gives the impression of a less personal space than the teen room.

Usually, one or more TOWs are present in the Teens room, either counseling clients, making follow-up phone calls, or catching up on some of the
endless paperwork necessitated by the clinic or the research project. Blanca,
the coordinating TOW, is always in and out supervising the TOWs and
counseling her own clients. She is the primary person responsible for the
day-to-day supervision of the TOWs and making sure the project runs
smoothly. Each month one of the TOWs is assigned to postpartum ward
outreach and has primary responsibility for visiting the new mothers on the
postpartum ward after delivery. She then adds those teens she has interviewed to her caseload. The newly delivered mothers are housed four to a
room on the ward. Since there are no telephones or televisions in the hospital rooms, visitors are frequently a welcome break.

In the clinic, the TOWs see the teen clients on both an appointment and
a walk-in basis. Only teen clients are allowed to be seen as walk-ins. During
a typical clinic visit, the TOWs provide counseling, education, and referrals;
perform routine procedures (blood pressure, urine tests, pregnancy tests,
etc.); consult with practitioners; and coordinate health care for their client,
often literally walking them through the system. The TOWs are responsible
for all their own follow-up and paperwork, and time must be scheduled to
allow for this. Telephone follow-up is the most troublesome because of the
difficulty of finding a free line during most of the day. Late afternoon seems
to be the best time to find free telephone lines, but may not be the best time
for follow-up with teens.

The TOWs are also called upon to help out in the regular clinic when staff
is short or more patients than usual show up for their appointments. Since a
large amount of in-kind support from the clinic was necessary for this project, and both the clinic and the Teen Project are administered by the clinic
administrator, there is a natural tendency to view the "special treatment" of
the teens as a luxury on days when the clinic is overcrowded or staff is short.
The TOWs are pulled into regular care to fill the gap, and this often puts
them behind in their own follow-up work with the research project.

This situation has led to some antagonism between the Teen Project staff
and the regular staff and to some ambivalence among the TOWs with respect
to their role. The TOWs are seen as "special" and privileged within the overall clinic system. They have a special room (the regular counselors are in one
big room with dividers) and more privacy. The teen clients are given priority
for health care even if they are late or do not have an appointment. The
TOWs' workloads appear to be lighter than those of counselors in the adult
clinic because they are allowed so much more time with teen clients (they
see fewer patients). The time involved in follow-up and paperwork required

by the project is not well understood, despite in-service presentations about the project. This uneasiness between the counselors in regular care and the TOWs was frequently a cause for concern, and many staff meetings addressed this issue. In part it seems to be a manifestation of the usual antagonism between research and patient care in any clinic setting, but also stems from the greater prestige attached to the TOW role. There was also a philosophical division between staff members who thought teen clients needed and deserved special treatment and those who thought they should not be coddled but should take responsibility for themselves and act like adults. All this made for particularly interesting and difficult employee relationships.

There were several other project staff who used the Teens room, including a research assistant who entered the data into the computer. There were two data entry persons over the course of the project; both were male Korean American university students and were computer science majors. They were extremely conscientious, and very few data entry errors were found despite very little supervision. Since they came during the evenings and weekends so as not to disrupt clinic hours, the coordinating TOW supervised their work, although sometimes my work schedule overlapped with theirs. There were also two other research assistants who were female public health master's students. They abstracted medical records for the project evaluation, and both used data from this project for their master's theses. The students came as their schedules permitted but usually during nonpeak hours, as clinic space was always at a premium when patients were present. During the Hewlett Project, I would also use this room about once or twice a week, supervising the overall project, managing and analyzing the data, answering questions, and writing reports and new proposals. I was also able to observe unobtrusively the interactions between the teens and the TOWs. Often, I encouraged the TOWs to probe for further information with a teen. This was possible because over the course of a clinic visit the teen would be in and out of the counseling room several times—when she arrived, before seeing the clinician, and after her exam. It was also occasionally possible for the research staff to use the work-station area adjacent to the Teens, but this area was used primarily by the practitioners for charting.

I would often stay in the evening after clinic hours to work when things were more quiet and peaceful. About once a month, one or more of the TOWs would stay late to talk about the project, specific clients, or problems with the data collection instruments. Some of our sessions would last several hours, especially if we got into an interesting topic such as abortion or the responsibilities of fathers to their children in Latino and American culture. Sometimes we would chat with a teen who was waiting for her ride home, or simply share current experiences, problems, hopes, and fears. Most of the ethnographic material, aside from the longitudinal case files, comes from these informal situations.

## The Research Team

### The TOWs

It is important to provide a characterization of the TOWs and the high-risk case manager, who was present during the first year of the project, because so much of the information reported in this study comes from their work, their comments, and their reactions to my interpretation of the data. In addition, as with most case-management programs, success with teens depends on the personalities of the staff and their ability to understand and work with teens. There were five TOWs over the three years of the project, three of whom remained for the full three years. All of them are Mexican American, bilingual, and bicultural. They all became role models for the young women in the program. They have been exceptionally dedicated and hard-working. They have all succeeded in overcoming the obstacles of being born into low socioeconomic status and have come back to the community to try to give something back and to make a difference there. The teens in their caseloads developed a considerable respect for and attachment to them, as did I.

Blanca, who was the head TOW and in her thirties, was herself a teenage mother and delivered her two children, a boy and a girl (now teenagers themselves), in the hospital where she now works helping young mothers avoid a subsequent pregnancy and helping them to see that they have options and choices in their lives. Blanca is the "mother" TOW, the kind of person who is always taking in strays, taking care of everyone, giving everybody the benefit of the doubt, and looking for the good in each person. She is eternally optimistic.

Blanca's mother came to the United States from Mexico with her first husband, whom she was forced by her family to marry. She later divorced and then met and married Blanca's father. Blanca is bilingual and bicultural and considers herself to be Mexican American. She grew up in the Estrada Courts housing projects in East L.A. Her mother divorced Blanca's father in 1956, and she now lives with her fourth husband, Blanca's stepfather, in South Gate, a nicer suburb about eleven miles from East L.A. Blanca has five half-siblings.

Blanca became pregnant with her first child in high school and married the father of her child. They had another child while she was completing school requirements to graduate. She and her husband were divorced after their second child was born, and to date she has not remarried. Blanca completed high school and received training as a family planning counselor. She has worked in family planning for eleven years.

Blanca and I worked together in the early 1980s at UCLA's family planning clinic as family planning counselors when I was going to school at UCLA. I have known her for almost fifteen years. After I became involved with the LAC-USC Family Planning Clinic, I tried for two years to convince Blanca to come to work with the Teen Project there, and I finally "stole" her away from UCLA (much to the chagrin of the clinic administrator, who recognized Blanca's abilities as well) to become the head TOW. She is a bright, energetic, articulate woman whose skills go far beyond her academic training. She is an especially good teacher and listener, and thus, is very good with teens. She also has a gift for understanding people, particularly children and adolescents. I have learned more about people, childrearing, and life from Blanca than, perhaps, from any other person I know. Her ambition is to go to college, after her children finish high school, and to specialize in preschool education.

Carmen, in her thirties, a bilingual bicultural Mexican American, has worked in family planning for ten years. Carmen was born in Mexico and grew up in Los Angeles, and lives in a very traditional Mexican family. She has ten brothers and sisters. Only one of her sisters was a teen mother. She is engaged to be married. Carmen took care of one of her sister's sons for seven years and only recently has her sister been able to take him to live with her. Carmen specializes in counseling HIV-positive[7] teens and adult women regarding family planning in conjunction with the HIV clinic at the hospital. Carmen has a patience and calmness that puts teens at ease. She is thorough, dependable, and nonjudgmental. She is the most quiet and private of the TOWs, perhaps the reason I know less about her than the others.

Lorinda, in her twenties, is the youngest of the TOWs. She grew up in Central Los Angeles and had her first child at age 14. She had a difficult time before she married the baby's father when their first son was 7 years old. They now have two boys. Lorinda finished high school and began working in family planning in 1988. She transferred from the regular clinic to the Teen Project when it began in 1989. Lorinda went through her second pregnancy and delivery during the time she worked for the Teen Project. She and her husband recently bought a house in Pico Rivera, a middle-class Latino community in L.A. Lorinda has been a special role model for the teens in the program. She represents to them the possibilities in their lives. Lorinda is also very much involved in counseling HIV-positive and high-risk women and recently completed training to be an HIV testing counselor. Lorinda has an inner strength and patience that I expect is comforting to the teen mothers in the program. It has always been comforting to me. She has an exceptional ability to empathize with their problems and listen to what they say. Lorinda wants to go to college and become a nurse and has started taking courses part-time.

Alicia, in her thirties, is Blanca's half-sister and worked with the Teen Project for two years before taking another job in the same clinic with the regular adult patient population. She is married and had two school-age daughters at the time she was with the project. Alicia was the "tough love" TOW. She always encouraged the teens to take responsibility for their lives. She left the project to take a more stable, county-funded position.[8]

América, in her twenties, replaced Alicia in 1991. She was in college majoring in social work at the time she took the job as part of an internship requirement for graduation. América grew up in East L.A. and has three siblings. Two of her younger sisters were teen mothers and had participated in the early years of the Teen Project prior to the Hewlett grant. She is the only one of the TOWs who has a college degree. She was married in the fall of 1991 and lives with her husband in Alhambra. América is beautiful, and she is the most fashion conscious of the group. Many of the Mexican American teens like this and relate to it. She represents a somewhat different role model, that of a young, upwardly mobile, college-educated professional Latina. She has taken over the high-risk caseload (i.e., involved with gangs and drugs, sexually or physically abused, medical problems of self or baby, extreme poverty, under age 15). América is a bright, thoughtful young woman who brings her expertise in social work to the program. She would like to complete her M.S.W.

### The High-risk Case Manager

Jorge, in his twenties, has a master's degree in social psychology and was part of the Teen Project until 1990, when the funding for the High-risk Case Management program provided by the California Community Foundation ended. Jorge served as the high-risk manager in the clinic for two years. He grew up in the "Jungle," that part of downtown Los Angeles west of the USC campus and Exposition Park. It is a mixed African American and Latino neighborhood northwest of South Central L.A. where the May 1992 riots in response to the Rodney King verdict took place. Jorge had worked with drug abusers and gang-involved male youth before coming to our project. There was considerable speculation among the staff and the medical director of the clinic about whether a young, single Latino male was the appropriate choice to be a case manager for the teen mothers, but any reservations were quickly overcome by the good response from the young women. He provided a positive male role model, very different from most of the men with whom they had been involved. Here was a handsome, young Latino man who respected education, and who respected women's rights. He encouraged them to go back to school, to think for themselves, and to question traditional male/female role relationships that tended to constrain their ability to become independent. Because of his previous work with drug-abusing teens, he was particularly adept at "connecting" with the drug-abusing teen mothers, and was able to see through their "scams." He also helped the TOWs by teaching them how to avoid dependency relationships with the teens in their case-loads. When the project ended, he was sorely missed.

### The Researcher, Pam

In this section I try to provide an account of myself, to present my biases as I see them, to describe my role in the field situation, and to provide some personal background.

First, I am an Anglo American in my forties, the eldest of two daughters from a loving, working-class, midwestern family. My family all immigrated from Sweden and Denmark in the early part of this century. My mother was first generation born in the United States, and my father second generation. I am married and have one child. I went through university on scholarships and worked part-time or full-time the entire twenty-odd years of my schooling. This includes doctorates in two disciplines: one academic, theoretical, holistic, qualitative—anthropology; the other scientific, pragmatic, quantitative, and a "helping profession"—public health. I often joke about being bidisciplinary, but I think it helps me to understand, at least a little, the phenomenon of biculturalism. I never feel completely at home in either of the disciplines in which I have been trained, but value the contribution of both to my scholarship. In this book, I try to integrate my two disciplines and their research methodologies to provide a comprehensive understanding of the Latina teenage pregnancy experience in Los Angeles.

As I became increasingly educated and began working as a professional, I had to learn appropriate patterns of upper-middle-class behavior, which were different from those of my family of origin. While I have learned to be "bi-class," I do not feel completely comfortable in either one and must "switch codes" depending on who I am with at the time. I suspect this also helps me to understand the experience of biculturalism, acculturation, and culture conflict between generations among immigrants.

My theoretical bias tends toward a biosocial interpretation of human behavior in environmental context. I think of a research question or problem as a diamond with many facets. Each of the facets provides a different understanding of the problem based on different theoretical interpretations (e.g., feminist, ecological, political, biological, psychological, cultural, etc.).

The real meaning lies in them all, perhaps a sum of all, perhaps more than the sum.

I do research that addresses contemporary social problems, and I apply the results in programs aimed at social betterment. I think it is imperative to work in partnership with the community through all phases of program design and implementation. I like being a part of all phases of applied social research: problem definition, research, intervention, evaluation, and policy recommendations.

Finally, I believe our society has a long way to go before we will have gender and racial equality, goals toward which I strive. I also believe that women must have the ultimate choice in decisions about childbearing, and I am a strong believer in civil liberties.

I came to my work with Latino adolescents in Los Angeles through my work in public health. As a public health student, I developed a strong interest in teenage pregnancy and childbearing and in adolescent risk-taking behavior (use of drugs/alcohol, nonuse of contraception, seat belt use). I became aware of the paucity of information on Latino teens, a growing ethnic group in Los Angeles County. I had studied the ethnology of Latin America as a student in anthropology, but not that of Latinos in the United States. Before becoming involved with Latinos in Los Angeles I had done research in Guatemala, Mexico, Panama, and Peru. I began learning about Latinos in the United States in the library and moved to the community, where it has taken many years to overcome suspicions about an Anglo researcher working with Latinos. I value the friendships I have developed with the Latinas with whom I have worked most closely. Only with time and effort will Angelenos be able to overcome the fears and prejudices that keep us racially and ethnically segregated.

I have never lived in East L.A. The barriers to neighborhood integration are real enough in Los Angeles as in other major cities. Like many other Anglos, I do not often move about in East L.A. neighborhoods unless I am accompanied by Latino friends. My friends always caution me about the dangers of being a foreigner, not necessarily an Anglo, in many neighborhoods. Fear, prejudice, poverty, drugs, and random gang violence are all too real in inner-city America, and they help to maintain racially, ethnically, and socioeconomically segregated neighborhoods.

Being in the Medical Center was easy because I had a defined role there, and it was "neutral" territory for local gangs, at least most of the time. There, to the patients and clients, I was just another Anglo "doctor, researcher, social worker, or nurse," not an intruder. To the family planning clinic staff and administrators, I had something to offer. I wrote the grants that provided the funding for the teen pregnancy prevention program and provided the research and evaluation skills necessary for the research project. From the point of view of the administration, the project was important. It was a model program for Latino pregnancy prevention, something to enhance public image. It was also good for the family planning clinic, which was always fighting for survival within the hospital system. From my point of view, I was both providing a service for teen mothers and, I hoped, influencing their lives for the better. I have received much more from the people with whom I worked than I have been able to return. I hope this book will contribute positively to the health and well-being of the young Latina women whom I have come to respect and admire for their courage and resourcefulness in taking on the responsibilities of motherhood.

The Teen Project was designed to test an intervention to delay rapid repeat pregnancy and was implemented exclusively in a medical setting. It is a logical extension of the medicalization of teenage pregnancy, which is primarily a socioeconomic problem, albeit with an important medical aspect. It was developed by Anglo health care professionals and implemented by the counselors and social workers, all of whom were Mexican American. The hospital setting shaped the project by providing the immediate physical and social context in which it was implemented. While it allowed contact with many Latina teen mothers, it also limited the type of contact possible. The hospital was located in East L.A., a center of Latino culture and large, recent immigration. The hospital was part of the L.A. County health system, a system that was beginning to feel the financial stresses that became so apparent in 1995. L.A. County was affected by the broader state and national policies regarding immigration and health care for the poor. All of these levels, from the microlevel of the Teen Project to the macrolevel issues of health care and immigration policy, provide the context for Latino teenage pregnancy in East L.A.

## CHAPTER FIVE

# The Latina Teen Mothers

The Hewlett Project collected detailed longitudinal data on project cases that allow in-depth description of the young women and the context in which they became mothers. The information presented in these next chapters is based on the 173 young women who were cases (i.e., clients of the program) and received the intensive contraceptive case-management follow-up (outlined in Chapter 3), and who had been interviewed in the hospital within twenty-four hours of the birth of their child.[1] All information reported in this chapter is based on the teens' self-report at the time of the postpartum interview except for the information on birth outcome, which was abstracted from medical records. Supporting information from interviews with TOWs and teen mothers over the course of the project is also used. Real case studies are included, using pseudonyms, only when there is no possible means of identifying the actual person. Some of the cases are fictitious in the sense that they are an amalgamation of several cases to protect individuals who might be identified by disclosure of their particular history.

## Situating the Hewlett Teens
## in the Latino Population

The teen mothers I describe are not representative of all Latina teen mothers in Los Angeles County or in California. They are poor, inner-city Latinas using the L.A. County health system. They reside primarily in the areas surrounding the hospital, which are immigrant dominated and poverty stricken. Nor are they representative of all teens who deliver at Women's Hospital. The family planning clinic draws patients from barrios surrounding the hospital and from among high-risk women who deliver at the hospital. Thus, these young mothers are likely to be at higher obstetric risk than the general population of teens aged 17 and under delivering at the hospital.

Table 5.1 presents information on demographic variables, prenatal care, and low birth weight for three groups of teen mothers aged 17 and under.

The first column presents information from the 1986–1987 postpartum ward surveys, the second column for the 1989–1991 Hewlett cases, and the third for postpartum ward surveys implemented in 1992–1994. The time periods of the ward surveys bracket that of the Hewlett Project.[2] The proportion foreign-born in all three groups is similar, ranging from 83% in the most recent ward survey to 90% in the Hewlett case group.[3] The proportion residing in the United States five or fewer years is almost identical, about three-fifths for all groups, as is the proportion who are Mexican born, 65%–67%. Spanish language preference is slightly higher among the Hewlett cases and the most recent delivery cohort, reflecting the influx of immigrants into the central city in the 1980s. Proportions of teens who had already had a prior child (13%–17%) and were in school when they became pregnant (37%–40%) are also similar. The proportion who planned their pregnancy was similar among the 1986–1987 group (34%) and the Hewlett cases (37%), but higher (58%) for the most recent 1992–1994 delivery cohort.

The most prominent differences between the Hewlett cases and the two delivery cohorts are related to age and obstetric risk. The Hewlett cases have a slightly greater proportion aged 15 and under and a lower proportion living with the baby's father. The Hewlett cases also have a greater proportion with late or no prenatal care and a greater proportion delivering low birth weight infants. These differences are consistent with the recruitment of teens with higher obstetric risk factors (i.e., young maternal age, no prenatal care, medical complications) into the Hewlett Project. In addition, the younger age of the Hewlett participants is probably related to the lower proportion living with the baby's father, since young teens (12–15 years old) tend not to form stable unions. These young mothers are actually quite similar to the population of Latina teens delivering at the hospital except for their higher obstetric risk.

The teen mothers described here, then, are a recent-immigrant, inner-city group who, nevertheless, make up a significant proportion of the Los Angeles population. Thus, adolescent childbearing among this group will have an important impact on L.A. and is of special interest to those interested in the Latino experience in California.

### Characteristics of Teen Mothers

#### Country of Birth, Language, and Acculturation

From previous work in the clinic it was clear that the Teen Project was not dealing with a homogeneous Latino population. First, there were differences in length of residence in the United States and language affiliation for

Table 5.1.    Characteristics of Latina Teen Mothers 17 Years of Age and Under at LAC-USC Women's and Children's Hospital

|  | Ward Surveys 1986–1987 $N = 1017$ | | Hewlett Cases 1989–1991 $N = 173$ | | Ward Surveys 1992–1994 $N = 1293$ | |
|---|---|---|---|---|---|---|
| Variable | N | % | N | % | N | % |
| Country of Birth | | | | | | |
| United States | 153 | 15 | 17 | 10 | 219 | 16 |
| Mexico | 669 | 67 | 112 | 65 | 831 | 65 |
| Central America | 187 | 19 | 43 | 25 | 236 | 19 |
| El Salvador | * | * | 27 | 16 | 122 | 10 |
| Other Latin | * | * | 16 | 9 | 114 | 9 |
| Total foreign-born | 856 | 85 | 155 | 90 | 1067 | 83 |
| = < 5 years in U.S. | 523 | 61 | 105 | 62 | 805 | 63 |
| Language | | | | | | |
| Spanish | 514 | 50 | 107 | 62 | 809 | 63 |
| Bilingual | 451 | 45 | 52 | 30 | 453 | 35 |
| English | 47 | 5 | 14 | 8 | 19 | 2 |
| Age = < 15 years | 148 | 21 | 49 | 28 | 279 | 22 |
| Partner age = < 20 years | 347 | 36 | 68 | 41 | 436 | 35 |
| > 1 child | 168 | 17 | 27 | 15 | 168 | 13 |
| In school | 394 | 40 | 61 | 37 | 478 | 38 |
| Planned pregnancy | 351 | 34 | 62 | 37 | 738 | 58 |
| Live with partner | 680 | 62 | 89 | 53 | 801 | 62 |
| Prenatal Care | | | | | | |
| 1st trimester | 416 | 42 | 44 | 26 | 599 | 52 |
| No care | 109 | 11 | 51 | 30 | 106 | 8 |
| Low birth weight | 88 | 8 | 31 | 18 | 115 | 9 |

* Item not on survey

the group. These were crosscut by cultural identification with country of birth and ethnic or cultural subgroups. In this sample, 90% of the teens were foreign-born (see Table 5.1). Mexico was most frequently reported as country of birth (65%). El Salvador was second (16%), Guatemala third (5%), Nicaragua fourth (3%), and 1% were from other Latin American countries. Only 17 teens (10%) were born in the United States.

Over half of these young mothers (62%) had lived in the United States five or fewer years (mean length of residence = 5.7, $s$ = 5.8 years), and over half (62%) preferred to speak Spanish (see Table 5.2). Thirty percent were bilingual, and 8% preferred English. Language preference was asked by the TOW before beginning the interview on the postpartum ward and indicates the language in which the teen conversed most comfortably.

There was a significant amount of overlap between country of birth and ethnic self-identification (see Table 5.2). Ninety-eight percent of those born

Table 5.2. Country of Birth, Language, and Years in United States for Hewlett Project Participants

| Variable | Total N | Total % | English Speakers N | English Speakers % | Spanish Speakers N | Spanish Speakers % | U.S. N | U.S. % | Mexico N | Mexico % | Central America N | Central America % |
|---|---|---|---|---|---|---|---|---|---|---|---|---|
| **Country of Birth (N = 172)** | | | | | | | | | | | | |
| U.S.A. | 17 | 10 | 16 | 24 | 1 | 1 | 17 | 100 | — | — | — | — |
| Mexico | 112 | 65 | 38 | 58 | 74 | 69 | — | — | 112 | 100 | — | — |
| Central America | 43 | 25 | 12 | 18 | 31 | 30 | — | — | — | — | 43 | 100 |
| El Salvador | 27 | 16 | 11 | 17 | 16 | 15 | — | — | — | — | 27 | 63 |
| Guatemala | 9 | 5 | 0 | — | 9 | 9 | — | — | — | — | 9 | 21 |
| Nicaragua | 5 | 3 | 0 | — | 5 | 5 | — | — | — | — | 5 | 12 |
| Other* | 2 | 1 | 1 | 2 | 1 | 1 | — | — | — | — | 2 | 5 |
| **Language Preferred (N = 173)†** | | | | | | | | | | | | |
| English | 14 | 8 | 14 | 21 | — | — | 6 | 35 | 7 | 6 | 1 | 2 |
| Bilingual | 52 | 30 | 52 | 79 | — | — | 10 | 59 | 31 | 28 | 11 | 26 |
| Spanish | 107 | 62 | — | — | 107 | 100 | 1 | 6 | 74 | 66 | 31 | 72 |
| **Years in United States (N = 170)** | | | | | | | | | | | | |
| 1 or less | 79 | 47 | 4 | 6 | 75 | 71 | — | — | 62 | 56 | 17 | 40 |
| 2–5 | 26 | 15 | 6 | 9 | 20 | 19 | — | — | 13 | 12 | 13 | 30 |
| >5 | 65 | 38 | 55 | 85 | 10 | 10 | 17 | 100 | 35 | 32 | 13 | 30 |
| Mean | 5.66 | | 11.31 | | 2.16 | | 15.94 | | 4.70 | | 4.05 | |
| s | 5.75 | | 4.90 | | 2.57 | | 0.75 | | 5.31 | | 3.39 | |
| Range | 1–17 | | 1–17 | | 1–16 | | 1–17 | | 1–17 | | 1–12 | |
| **Self-Identification (N = 172)** | | | | | | | | | | | | |
| American | 2 | 1 | 1 | 2 | 1 | — | 1 | — | 0 | — | 1 | 2 |
| Mex-Amer | 17 | 10 | 16 | 24 | 1 | — | 15 | 88 | 2 | 2 | 0 | — |
| Mexican | 115 | 67 | 38 | 58 | 77 | 73 | 1 | 6 | 110 | 98 | 4 | 9 |
| Salvadoran | 25 | 15 | 10 | 15 | 15 | 14 | — | — | — | — | 25 | 58 |
| Guatemalan | 9 | 5 | 0 | — | 9 | 8 | — | — | — | — | 9 | 21 |
| Other | 4 | 2 | 1 | 1 | 3 | 3 | — | — | — | — | 4 | 9 |

s = standard deviation

* Belize, Honduras

† U.S./Mexico: N = 172

in Mexico identified themselves as Mexican; 94% of the U.S.-born identified themselves as Mexican American or American; and 88% of those born in Central America indicated they identified with their country of birth.

Among the Mexican-origin group, self-identifying as either Mexican or Mexican American seemed to be related to the number of years a teen had resided in the United States and her language preference. For example,

*María, age 15*

María was born in Mexico but came to the United States when she was six months old and received all her schooling here. She is bilingual and considers herself to be Mexican American.

*Claudia, age 17*

Claudia was born in the United States, has lived here all her life, speaks English, and also considers herself to be Mexican American.

*Aurora, age 17*

Aurora, on the other hand, immigrated to the United States from Mexico less than a year before the birth of her child, speaks only Spanish, and has never been to school in the United States. She self-identifies as Mexican.

*Carina, age 15*

Carina was born in Nicaragua and has lived in the United States for three years. She prefers Spanish but also speaks fair English and has been to school in the United States. She considers herself Nicaraguan.

Only two of the teens in the sample (one born in Guatemala and one born in the United States) considered themselves to be American, suggesting the strength and persistence of identification with country of birth.

The study did not use a formal measure of acculturation, but did include several variables that appear to be important indicators of level of acculturation for Latino teenagers in the Southwest. These include preferred language, length of residence in the United States, and ethnic self-identification, which together have been shown to account for much of the variation in acculturation (Becerra and de Anda 1984; Erickson 1988; Marin et al. 1987; Scrimshaw et al. 1987). Since preferred language captured most of the differences in these other variables for this sample, it was chosen to summarize acculturation level.[4] Spanish as the preferred language was virtually synonymous with foreign birth (99% of Spanish speakers), recent entry into the United States (71% had resided in the United States one year or less with a mean length of residence of 2.2, $s = 2.6$ years), and self-identification with the country of origin (not shown in table).

The bilingual teens and those who preferred English were born predominantly outside the United States (75%) but had a longer period of residence in the United States (85% had resided in the United States more than five years and had a mean length of residence of 11.3, $s = 4.9$ years). They were also more likely to self-identify as Mexican American (24%) than Spanish speakers (1%), but the majority identified as Mexican (58%).[5] Collapsing these last two language preferences together allows for more robust quantitative comparisons, but it might mask differences between bilingual and predominantly English-speaking teens. Unfortunately, the size of the group preferring English is just too small ($N = 14$) to consider separately. Thus, the English-speaking group includes both English-speaking and bilingual teens.

The English-speaking group probably represents a continuum of acculturation levels, but the teens in this group have shared an acculturative or bicultural process in the United States through long-term residence, school, language, and peer socialization. Similarity of experience within the Spanish-speaking group, however, cannot be as easily assumed. It is well known that Latino populations in the United States show a great deal of variation in macrolevel variables such as education level, fertility, and income (Bean and Tienda 1987). The Spanish-speaking group in this sample is composed of teens primarily from Mexico and Central America.[6] Each of the countries involved has its own history and culture despite overall similarities in language, religion, and status as former colonies of Spain.

In addition, the history of migration to the United States from these two areas is quite different. There is a long history of immigration from Mexico primarily for economic reasons, and historically most immigrants from Mexico have tended to be from lower socioeconomic classes, frequently from rural areas. There is also a considerable fluidity of population movement between the southwestern United States and Mexico. Many families have relatives in both countries, and visiting Mexico, sometimes for extended periods, is not uncommon. In fact, one of the threats parents often use with their teenage children is to send them to live with relatives in Mexico if they do not behave.

On the other hand, Central American migration to the United States is a relatively recent phenomenon. It has occurred largely in response to the devastating civil wars in El Salvador, Guatemala, and Nicaragua over the past two decades. Many families have sent their children to the United States one at a time as finances allowed before finally migrating themselves. Many have come as political refugees and may also have experienced incarceration, terror, torture, and death of loved ones at home. Others have come as a result of deteriorating economic conditions in their homeland. Thus, many Central

Table 5.3.  Age, Pregnancy History, and Pregnancy Planning

| Variable | Total | | English Speakers | | Spanish Speakers | | U.S. | | Mexico | | Central America | |
|---|---|---|---|---|---|---|---|---|---|---|---|---|
| | N | % | N | % | N | % | N | % | N | % | N | % |
| Age (N = 173)† | | | | | | | | | | | | |
| 13 | 4 | 2 | 2 | 3 | 2 | 2 | 0 | — | 4 | 4 | 0 | — |
| 14 | 14 | 8 | 7 | 11 | 7 | 7 | 0 | — | 10 | 9 | 4 | 9 |
| 15 | 31 | 18 | 17 | 26 | 14 | 13 | 5 | 29 | 21 | 19 | 5 | 12 |
| 16 | 57 | 33 | 20 | 30 | 37 | 35 | 8 | 47 | 32 | 29 | 16 | 37 |
| 17 | 67 | 39 | 20 | 30 | 47 | 44 | 4 | 24 | 45 | 40 | 18 | 40 |
| Mean | 15.98 | | 15.74 | | 16.12 | | 15.94 | | 15.93 | | 16.12 | |
| s | 1.05 | | 1.10 | | 1.00 | | 0.75 | | 1.13 | | 0.96 | |
| Number of Pregnancies (N = 173)† | | | | | | | | | | | | |
| 1 | 135 | 78 | 50 | 76 | 85 | 79 | 13 | 77 | 85 | 76 | 36 | 84 |
| 2 | 31 | 18 | 14 | 21 | 17 | 16 | 4 | 24 | 21 | 19 | 6 | 14 |
| 3 | 7 | 4 | 2 | 3 | 5 | 5 | 0 | — | 6 | 5 | 1 | 2 |
| Mean | 1.26 | | 1.27 | | 1.25 | | 1.24 | | 1.30 | | 1.19 | |
| s | 0.52 | | 0.51 | | 0.53 | | 0.44 | | 0.56 | | 0.45 | |
| Number of Births (N = 173) | | | | | | | | | | | | |
| 1 | 146 | 84 | 55 | 83 | 91 | 85 | 15 | 88 | 90 | 80 | 40 | 93 |
| 2 | 23 | 13 | 9 | 14 | 14 | 13 | 2 | 12 | 18 | 16 | 4 | 7 |
| 3 | 4 | 2 | 2 | 3 | 2 | 2 | 0 | — | 4 | 4 | 0 | — |
| Mean | 1.18 | | 1.20 | | 1.17 | | 1.12 | | 1.23 | | 1.06 | |
| s | 0.44 | | 0.47 | | 0.43 | | 0.33 | | 0.50 | | 0.26 | |
| Pregnancy Planned (N = 166) | | | | | | | | | | | | |
| Yes | 62 | 37 | 18 | 28 | 44 | 43 | 4 | 24 | 40 | 37 | 18 | 44 |
| No/OK* | 79 | 48 | 41 | 63 | 38 | 38 | 11 | 65 | 55 | 51 | 13 | 32 |
| No | 25 | 15 | 6 | 9 | 19 | 19 | 2 | 12 | 13 | 12 | 10 | 24 |
| Boyfriend/Baby's Father Wanted Pregnancy (N = 161) | | | | | | | | | | | | |
| Yes | 82 | 51 | 28 | 45 | 54 | 55 | 7 | 44 | 56 | 52 | 19 | 50 |
| No | 47 | 29 | 19 | 30 | 28 | 29 | 7 | 44 | 31 | 29 | 9 | 24 |
| DK** | 32 | 20 | 16 | 25 | 16 | 16 | 2 | 12 | 20 | 19 | 10 | 26 |

s = standard deviation       †U.S./Mexico: N = 172       * Pregnancy not planned, but teen felt it was "OK" now       ** Don't know or no relationship

Americans do not see return to their country of origin as an option. Unlike the Mexican migrants, the Central Americans tend to view themselves as permanent immigrants. Also unlike Mexican migrants, many were middle class in their country of birth.

Because of the possible differences introduced by level of acculturation (English speakers/Spanish speakers) and by area of origin (United States, Mexico, Central America), throughout this book comparisons will be made both by acculturation and cultural group (i.e., English/Spanish, United States/Mexico/Central America).

### Age, Parity, and Pregnancy Planning

The young women ranged from 13 to 17 years of age with a mean age of 16, $s = 1.05$ years (see Table 5.3). Over one-third (39%) were 17; 33% were 16; and 28% were under 16, with 10% under 15. The English speakers were slightly younger (about four months on average) than the Spanish speakers (mean age 15.7 vs. 16.1, $t = 2.2809$, $df = 127.5$, $p < .05$), but there were no differences in mean age among the three cultural groups.

Most of the teens in this sample had experienced only one pregnancy (78%), and most were having their first baby (84%). A sizable proportion (16%) were having their second or third child (see Table 5.3). There were no statistically significant differences between English and Spanish speakers nor among the cultural groups regarding number of pregnancies and births. There was a tendency for Mexicans to have higher parity, however, with 16% having their second child and 4% their third child compared to 12% of the U.S.-born and 7% of Central American teens having a second child. Neither of these last two groups had any teen mothers with more than two births. Only a small percentage (6%, or 10 teens) of the sample had had a previous spontaneous abortion (SAB), and three teens (2%) had had a prior therapeutic abortion (TAB).

Over one-third of the pregnancies to these young women (37%) had been planned; that is, the teen was actively trying to become pregnant (see Table 5.3).[7] While a third of the teens said they had definitely planned the pregnancy, slightly more than half (51%) indicated that the baby's father had wanted them to become pregnant.

In the course of the Teen Project there was only one Latina teen who had considered giving up her baby for adoption, a 12-year-old Central American girl. The TOWs helped her to arrange a private adoption to a Latino family in northern California, but at the last moment the girl's mother (i.e., the baby's grandmother) refused to sign the adoption papers. The 12-year-old was lost to follow-up after that.

Not surprisingly, teens who were married or living with their partners

Table 5.4.  Education (N = 173)

| Variable | Total | | English Speakers | | Spanish Speakers | | U.S. | | Mexico | | Central America | |
|---|---|---|---|---|---|---|---|---|---|---|---|---|
| | N | % | N | % | N | % | N | % | N | % | N | % |
| *Variable* | | | | | | | | | | | | |
| Mean grade completed at delivery (N = 169)* | | | | | | | | | | | | |
| Mean | 7.85 | | 8.79 | | 7.25 | | 8.71 | | 7.64 | | 8.02 | |
| s | 2.12 | | 1.40 | | 2.29 | | 1.90 | | 2.14 | | 2.14 | |
| Range | 1–12 | | 3–11 | | 1–12 | | 3–11 | | 1–11 | | 3–12 | |
| Attended school in United States (N = 159)† | | | | | | | | | | | | |
| Yes | 86 | 54 | 59 | 95 | 27 | 28 | 13 | 87 | 50 | 50 | 22 | 51 |
| No | 73 | 46 | 3 | 5 | 70 | 72 | 2 | 13 | 50 | 50 | 21 | 49 |
| In school when became pregnant (N = 164)‡ | | | | | | | | | | | | |
| Yes | 40 | 24 | 30 | 49 | 10 | 10 | 6 | 38 | 24 | 23 | 9 | 21 |
| Dropped out | 21 | 13 | 9 | 15 | 2 | 12 | 3 | 19 | 11 | 10 | 7 | 17 |
| No | 103 | 63 | 22 | 36 | 81 | 78 | 7 | 43 | 70 | 67 | 26 | 62 |
| Wants to return to school after baby is born (N = 164)‡ | | | | | | | | | | | | |
| No | 25 | 15 | 2 | 3 | 23 | 23 | 1 | 7 | 19 | 18 | 5 | 12 |
| Yes | 110 | 67 | 53 | 83 | 57 | 51 | 12 | 79 | 64 | 60 | 33 | 79 |
| Yes, but can't with baby | 22 | 13 | 6 | 9 | 16 | 16 | 1 | 7 | 18 | 17 | 3 | 7 |
| Yes, but partner won't allow | 7 | 4 | 3 | 5 | 4 | 4 | 1 | 7 | 5 | 5 | 1 | 2 |

s = standard deviation     * U.S./Mexico: N = 168     † U.S./Mexico: N = 158     ‡ U.S./Mexico: N = 163 were more likely to report having a planned pregnancy (52%) than either those who had no relationship with the father after the birth (16%) or those who were still involved with the baby's father but were not living together (40%) (chi-square = 18.864, $df = 2$, $p < .0001$). Teens who were married or living with their partners were also more likely to report that the baby's father wanted the pregnancy (76%) than those who had no relationship with him after the birth (16%) or those who were still involved but not living together (50%; chi-square = 48.695, $df = 2$, $p < .0001$).

English-speaking teens were less likely than Spanish speakers to have planned their pregnancies (chi-square = 4.258, $df = 1$, $p < .05$), but there was no difference among the three cultural groups regarding the proportions of teens who said their pregnancies were planned. Over one-third of all these young mothers had planned their pregnancies, and 48% welcomed them after the fact. National estimates indicate that only 26% of all teen pregnancies are planned, 49% of those among married teens and only 14% of those among unmarried teens (Alan Guttmacher Institute 1981). Since a large proportion of the teens in this sample were married or living with their partners (53%; see Table 5.5), the overall percentage of teens who had planned their pregnancies was higher than that of the national overall percentage, in which a larger proportion of teen mothers were unmarried. However, the percentages parallel national trends when relationship to the baby's father is taken into consideration.

### Education and Occupation

Over half (54%) of these young mothers had attended school in the United States (see Table 5.4), and English speakers were much more likely than Spanish speakers to have done so (95% vs. 28%; chi-square = 69.041, $df = 1$, $p < .0001$). Interestingly, about 3% of the U.S.-born teens indicated they had not attended school in the United States. This suggests that they might have lived in Mexico during their childhood. Alternatively, they may have been misrepresenting themselves as U.S.-born. The proximity of Tijuana and other border towns allows many extended families to live on both sides of the U.S.-Mexico border, and frequently families can live better on American salaries in Tijuana than in the United States. Unfortunately, we did not probe into this aspect of the young women's past lives.

The mean grade level completed by the respondents was 7.85, $s = 2.12$, about two years behind the average grade level expected for the mean age of this population (i.e., expected grade under the American system starting with kindergarten at age 5). English speakers had, on overage, about 1.5 more years of schooling than Spanish speakers (mean of 8.8 vs. 7.3; $t = 4.8894$, $df = 167$, $p < .00001$), but there was no difference in grade level completed by the three cultural groups. Nearly all (94%) indicated they could read and write in at least one language, and this was confirmed in the clinic when teens had to read and sign consent forms for medical treatment or contraception. While some teens had difficulty with the complicated language on the forms, there were only a few teens who were illiterate.

Interviews with the TOWs and some of the young mothers from Mexico suggest that there is a general feeling in Mexico that a primary school education is sufficient for females and that if a girl does not have a boyfriend by age 15 or 16, she is considered by her peers to be an "old maid." As a 16-year-old teen mother from Baja California noted, "Over there [in Mexico] if you're not *prometida* (engaged) by 15 they think there is something wrong with you." Another teen suggested that schooling beyond *primaria* (grades one through six) was expensive for those living in rural areas because they frequently had to travel to a larger town to enroll in the higher grade levels. This was considered a great expense, and if anyone in the family went to school it would be a boy and not a girl.

More than half (63%) of these young women were not attending school when they became pregnant, and about a third of those who were attending school said they had dropped out because of the pregnancy. A much greater proportion of Spanish (78%) than English speakers (36%) were not in school when they became pregnant, and a smaller proportion of English speakers dropped out (23%) due to pregnancy (vs. 55% of Spanish speakers; chi-square = 29.727, $df = 1$, $p < .0001$). Of the cultural groups, the U.S.-born had a higher proportion in school when they became pregnant than either of the foreign-born groups, although the relationship was not statistically significant. It is possible that the Spanish-speaking Latina mothers might have found more of an incompatibility between the roles of schoolgirl and wife-mother than their more acculturated sisters or than Anglo-American or African American teen mothers, who may have more support from family and friends to remain in school. This was only hinted at in comments made by teens regarding their perceptions of what their partners and family members expected of them after they became pregnant.

The same attitude was expressed by the teens themselves with respect to the idea of school return. When asked if they wanted to go back to school after the baby was born, the majority said yes (80% or more across all groups; see Table 5.4). However, a sizable proportion of those saying yes, about one-fifth overall, indicated that although they would like to return to school, their new responsibilities as mothers (and in many cases as housewives as well) did not allow this. Less than half thought it was likely that they actually would return to school.

Both family members and partners reinforced the mother-housewife role, as Elena notes:

> I'd like to go back to school, but my mother says that now that I have a baby I have to stay home and be a mother. It's my duty. I can't leave her [the baby], anyway, she's too little. Maybe when she gets older and can stay with my sister and her kids.

Similarly Ana says of her partner:

> Ay, he won't let me go back to school. He says I have to stay home and be a wife and mother now. That's what I'm supposed to do. He needs me there. I say "what about night school?" And he says, "OK, I can watch him at night," but then he won't do it when it gets down to it. He wants me home. He works all day—hard, you know—and he's tired. He wants me to make dinner and take care of the baby.

Jealousy on the part of the partner may also be a factor. Teens would often indicate that their partners watched their behavior closely, didn't like them to go out much, and wanted their wives/girlfriends at home. Sometimes this was extreme, as in the case of María.

### María, age 16

María had recently arrived from Mexico when she became involved with a 25-year-old Mexican man with whom she lives in a hotel room in downtown Los Angeles. María confided to a TOW that since she moved in with him he keeps her literally locked in their room and won't allow her to go out for any reason without him. He brings her everything she needs for the baby. He is also physically abusive, but María has no family in the United States and is here illegally. She is afraid to leave her only source of economic support.

Rather than keeping the teen a prisoner, as described in the case above, more often it was just a close watch by the partner and his family and friends, and often, too, by her own family. In the case of a gang-involved partner, the surveillance could sometimes take on frightening overtones, as Lupe explains:

> I couldn't go anywhere without him knowing where I was going. All his homeboys [other male gang members or would-be gang members from the neighborhood] would watch me, too. I couldn't get away from him. He knew my every move.

Lupe eventually went to Mexico for an extended visit to try to sever ties with her baby's father, a drug dealer. She told the TOWs that the baby was her reason for leaving behind the *chola* life. Scrimshaw (1978a) has discussed this close guarding of young wives as a typical pattern in Latin American societies. It is apparent that this pattern becomes elaborated in different ways in the United States. The young mothers seem both pleased and annoyed by this apparent show of affection, territoriality, and possession. Many, however, are resigned and express feelings of loneliness and confinement, particularly those who have been to school in the United States and are accustomed to a much freer lifestyle.

As indicated above, most of the young mothers do not think it is likely that they will return to school, and, in fact, the prospects for school return among young Latina teen mothers are not high (Fennelly 1993). In the short term, among the teens in this sample who remained in the program, only 10% to 15% returned to school during the year following the birth. Past experience with this population suggests that while the teens consistently reported wanting to go back to school, in most cases they found it impossible to return unless they found a school with child care on site or had family members willing to take over the child-care responsibilities.

These two options are less than realistic for this population. Los Angeles does have two public schools (Riley High and McAlister High) with six regional centers for pregnant and parenting teens that have on-site child-care facilities. These centers are spread throughout the (very large) school district, and the names on the waiting lists often number in the hundreds for twenty to thirty spaces. Demand outstrips supply, and teens who have not been in school for several years are not likely to have priority for placement in such programs.

Second, many of the teens who enter the Teen Project already live with their partner or live within female-headed households (62% do not have their own fathers in Los Angeles), leaving little opportunity for child care from their working mothers, who often rely on their own teenage daughters to care for their younger siblings. The broader literature on teenage childbearing strongly suggests that teen mothers who do not marry and who live with their own mothers consistently fare better economically over the long term than those who marry, because they tend to return to school, to prevent repeat births, and to find employment (Dryfoos 1982). However, these are the goals of a largely white, middle-class, health-professional population and may not be shared by different cultural groups. Moreover, the effect of living at home is a direct result of the heavy investment by the teen mother's own mother and other family members in terms of child care and the encouragement of school return. For reasons discussed above, these may not be realistic expectations in this low-income Latino population. That is, school may be less highly valued for females and seen as direct competition to what is perceived as the more important maternal role, and opportunities for school return are limited.

Because such a high proportion of teens had dropped out of school prior to becoming pregnant (63%), we were curious to learn more about how they had occupied their time and asked them what they had been doing before they became pregnant. The most common response was that they were simply staying at home "doing nothing/*nada*" (42%). About one-fifth (21%) were already "housewives/*amas de casa*." Another fifth were "taking care of children/*cuidando niños*" who were either not their own (14%) or their own (5%). Three examples from case materials illustrate:

### Sinamon, "doing nothing"

Sinamon is one example of a teen who was staying at home not doing much before or during her pregnancy except waiting to come to the United States to be with her husband. Sinamon is 16, married to a 28-year-old. Both are from Guatemala and speak Spanish. Sinamon arrived in the United States two months before delivering her child. She received no prenatal care in the United States. Her husband, who came before she did, started working at a new job the day of our interview with her. They live with some of her relatives. Her mother and father do not live in the United States. Sinamon completed ten years of schooling and her husband twelve years. At the postpartum interview she was planning to return to Guatemala, but she actually remained in the United States and continued in the program for over a year until she was finally lost to follow-up after a positive pregnancy test.

### Aurora, "a housewife"

Aurora is a 17-year-old Spanish-speaking teen who dropped out of school after eighth grade when she migrated with her family to the United States from Mexico. She did not enter school in the United States, and was living off and on with her 19-year-old boyfriend, Jorge, being a housewife. She was not trying to get pregnant but indicated that they had wanted a baby at some point. At the time of the birth she had not seen Jorge for several months and had moved in permanently with her aunt. She said she had not known anything about sex or birth control and was afraid when she found out she was pregnant.

### Inocencia, "baby-sitting"

Inocencia is 14 years old, a Spanish speaker from Mexico who has been in the United States for less than two years. She lives with the baby's father, Juan, and his family. Juan is 19 years old, completed third grade, and is employed as a cook. Inocencia completed sixth grade in Mexico. She was baby-sitting for relatives while she and Juan were trying to have a baby of their own. She wants another child in five years. They are both very happy about the baby and plan to marry.

A small percentage (10%) of the teens were working for wages, and another 9% gave some other response to the question. Most of those who worked were either clerical workers (18%), laborers (23%), or service workers (27%), according to the Hollingshead classification system. Laborers included workers in the garment industry or other light industries.

### Isabel, garment worker

Isabel, aged 17, is a Spanish-speaking recent immigrant from Mexico who had her first child at age 16 by a different man than the father of the child who brought her into our program. She was working in a garment factory when she met Luis, her present partner, who is 29 (twelve years older than Isabel) and has a steady job in the same garment factory where Isabel works. They are planning to marry and both had wanted this pregnancy. Isabel's first child lives with her own mother in Mexico.

Service workers included maids, food service workers, baby-sitters, and house cleaners. Large numbers of less educated and undocumented persons in Los Angeles are employed in these occupations. Undocumented women can easily find work cleaning or caring for children in private homes, and there is a huge demand for their labor among the middle class. The whole system is informal. Referral is by word of mouth and the pay is low, but threat of detection by the Immigration and Naturalization Service (INS) is also very low, making such positions appealing. The situation in Los Angeles is not dissimilar to that in many large Latin American cities, where the middle class relies on the informal and low-paid labor of the lower class to provide the support services (child care, cooking, and cleaning) that allow middle-class women the opportunity to work outside the home and increase or maintain their middle-class standard of living. Little is known about Latinas' participation in this informal labor sector and its effect on household income, fertility, partner relationships, and child care.

Although data were not collected regarding family income, all of the teens in this sample and their families were low income. The use of public assistance aside from Medi-Cal (California's Medicaid program) and WIC (the federal Women, Infants, and Children food supplementation program for pregnant and lactating women and children under three), however, was very low. At the postpartum interview, 99% of the teens were planning to rely on Medi-Cal to pay for the medical expenses related to the birth, and 40% were referred to the WIC program. Only three teens were referred to the Department of Human Services for Aid to Families with Dependent

Children (AFDC). This reflects two factors: (1) there are many teens who deliver babies at the hospital who are illegally in the United States and, therefore, not eligible for government assistance other than Medi-Cal and WIC; and (2) the Mexican population generally does not rely on public assistance. According to Jorge, the former high-risk case manager, there are two reasons for this. First, there is a general cultural bias against welfare dependency among Mexicans and Mexican Americans. People work and take pride in their ability to support their families even if they are poor. Blanca, the head TOW, told me that when she was a child growing up in the housing projects in East L.A. her mother used to tell her and her brothers and sisters to be proud. Although they were poor, they were loved, clean, had shoes, were getting an education, and had enough to eat. That was all that mattered.

Second, although families going through the amnesty process are allowed to receive state benefits for children born in the United States, they fear that availing themselves of this support might jeopardize their chances of approval. As Jorge told me:

> Although the babies are eligible for welfare, a lot of girls don't want to use it. You have to go for an interview for the amnesty process, and if they see you've been on welfare at all, they can make the process harder on you. So even though it's legal, the word is out. . . . Rosa just went off AFDC because of that. For my kids [cases] who've only been here two years and there's no way they're ever gonna [sic] be eligible [for amnesty under IRCA], I just tell them to go for it [AFDC]. Why suffer?

Thus, as Blanca summarizes:

> These teens and their partners are the working poor. They work long hours at low-paying jobs with no benefits and can barely manage the costs of the new baby. Even with WIC and Medi-Cal, the cost of diapers is not covered . . . then if there are other children, too . . . it's just too much.

### Relationship to Baby's Father

Overall, more than half (53%) of these young women were married or living with the baby's father (see Table 5.5). Sixteen percent were legally married. Spanish speakers (22%) were more likely to be married than English speakers (6%). Among the three cultural groups, none of the U.S.-born teens were married, compared to 20% of the Mexican-born and 12% of the Central American–born teens. The TOWs distinguished teens who were legally married from those who were living together in informal union by asking the date of the wedding. This was a very clever addition to the interview by the TOWs when, early on in the research, they had discovered a tendency among the teens to say they were married when they were

Table 5.5.    Relationship to Baby's Father

| Variable | Total | | English Speakers | | Spanish Speakers | | U.S. | | Mexico | | Central America | |
|---|---|---|---|---|---|---|---|---|---|---|---|---|
| | N | % | N | % | N | % | N | % | N | % | N | % |
| Relationship to Baby's Father (N = 169)* | | | | | | | | | | | | |
| Married | 27 | 16 | 4 | 6 | 23 | 22 | 0 | 0 | 22 | 20 | 5 | 12 |
| Live/w | 62 | 37 | 27 | 41 | 35 | 34 | 11 | 65 | 35 | 32 | 16 | 38 |
| Boyfriend | 21 | 12 | 16 | 24 | 5 | 5 | 3 | 18 | 11 | 10 | 6 | 14 |
| None | 59 | 35 | 19 | 29 | 40 | 39 | 3 | 18 | 41 | 38 | 15 | 36 |
| Partner's Age and Partner/Teen Age Differences (N = 168)** | | | | | | | | | | | | |
| Age of boyfriend | | | | | | | | | | | | |
| Mean | 21.08 | | 20.36 | | 21.53 | | 20.53 | | 20.85 | | 21.98 | |
| s | 3.59 | | 3.22 | | 3.75 | | 3.26 | | 3.47 | | 4.01 | |
| Range | 15–31 | | 15–31 | | 16–31 | | 16–29 | | 15–31 | | 16–31 | |
| Differences in ages (N = 168)** | | | | | | | | | | | | |
| Mean | 5.10 | | 4.63 | | 5.39 | | 4.59 | | 4.92 | | 5.85 | |
| s | 3.60 | | 3.23 | | 3.80 | | 3.55 | | 3.46 | | 4.01 | |
| Range | 0–16 | | 0–15 | | 0–16 | | 0–14 | | 0–16 | | 0–15 | |
| Partner's Grade and Partner/Teen Grade Differences (N = 104)† | | | | | | | | | | | | |
| Grade of boyfriend | | | | | | | | | | | | |
| Mean | 8.91 | | 10.10 | | 7.86 | | 9.80 | | 8.49 | | 9.39 | |
| s | 3.12 | | 2.37 | | 3.34 | | 2.73 | | 3.32 | | 2.68 | |
| Range | 1–16 | | 1–12 | | 2–16 | | 3–12 | | 1–16 | | 2–12 | |
| Difference in grades (N = 103)‡ | | | | | | | | | | | | |
| Mean | 0.86 | | 1.31 | | 0.46 | | 1.07 | | 0.63 | | 1.30 | |
| s | 2.84 | | 2.66 | | 2.97 | | 3.31 | | 2.93 | | 2.30 | |
| Range | -6–9 | | -6–6 | | -6–7 | | -6–9 | | -6–7 | | -6–5 | |
| Baby's Father's Preferred Language (N = 168)** | | | | | | | | | | | | |
| English | 15 | 9 | 11 | 18 | 4 | 4 | 2 | 12 | 10 | 9 | 3 | 7 |
| Bilingual | 50 | 30 | 33 | 52 | 17 | 16 | 7 | 41 | 26 | 24 | 16 | 40 |
| Spanish | 103 | 61 | 19 | 30 | 84 | 80 | 8 | 47 | 74 | 67 | 21 | 53 |

s = standard deviation    * U.S./Mexico: N = 168    ** U.S./Mexico: N = 167    † U.S./Mexico: N = 103    ‡ U.S./Mexico: N = 102 actually living together in informal union. When they asked when the teen and her partner had been married, the informal status of the union would be confided. One-third (37%) of the teen mothers were not married but were living with the baby's father. Thus, while about half of the teens in all groups had serious relationships with the fathers of their babies, the proportions who were legally married differed among them.

Another 12% of the young mothers reported they had a boyfriend-girlfriend relationship (5% of Spanish and 24% of English speakers). The U.S.-born teens were the most likely to report this type of relationship (18%) compared to about 10% of Mexican-born and 14% of Central American–born teens. The remaining third (35%) had no current relationship with the baby's father, and Spanish speakers and the foreign-born had slightly higher proportions having no relationship to the baby's father. Of those having no relationship, 31% indicated the baby's father was not in the United States, 24% simply said without further elaboration that there was no relationship, five teens (9%) were abandoned because of the pregnancy, four teens (7%) stated they had become pregnant as a result of rape, and three teens (5%) had not told the father about the pregnancy.

The mean age of the fathers was 21 years ($s = 3.59$) and ranged from 15 to 31 (see Table 5.5). On the average, the fathers were about five years ($s = 3.60$, range 0–16) older than the teens themselves. This age difference was highest among the Spanish speakers and among those born in Central America. The partners also had a mean of about one more year (mean = 0.86, $s = 2.84$) of schooling than the teens, although a lower proportion (40%) had been in school in the United States.

Although such wide age differences between teen mothers and their partners have been documented in national studies (Landry and Forrest 1995), the TOWs and I often spoke of what seemed to be the vast age differences between the teens and their partners. Each of the TOWs agreed that the age difference was really more than they would consider "right" or acceptable in their own culture, given that these teens were so young. Blanca, however, offered the explanation that "over there" [in Mexico] it was not so unusual. Marriages began earlier, and having a man who *"ya tiene su carrera"* (already has his career going) was considered preferable to marrying one who was not yet settled. Jorge gave another perspective on this when he told us about his father's counsel that he find a younger woman to marry so that he could "train her" to be a good wife. Both points of view are reminiscent of the stereotypical sex roles of the traditional dependent wife and mother and the husband and father who provides economically and protects his family.

The baby's father's language preference and country of birth closely paralleled those of the teens. Sixty-one percent were Spanish speakers, 30%

were bilingual, and 9% were English speakers. Similarly, 89% were foreign-born, with Mexico (64%) most frequently reported, followed by El Salvador (14%) and Guatemala (7%). Sixty-six percent of the teen mothers reported being born in the same country as the baby's father (80% of Spanish speakers but only 42% of English speakers).

It is worth noting here that the 16- and 17-year-old mothers were more likely than younger teens to be married or living with the baby's father (60% vs. 35%; chi-square = 9.741, $df = 2$, $p < .01$), and that the youngest teens (13–15 years old) were more likely (45%) than the older teens (31%) to have no current relationship with the baby's father or to be in an informal (boyfriend/girlfriend) relationship with him (20% vs. 9%).

Health care providers often say that with very young pregnant or parenting teens (under age 15) they tend to assume the girl has been raped, whether she indicates this or not. Certainly, having sex with an underage female constitutes statutory rape, and in the majority of cases (60%) the very young teens in this sample were involved with adult males (over age 18). The mean age difference between these youngest teens and their partners was 5.57 years ($s = 3.75$), and the mean age of their partners was 20.13 ($s = 3.75$, range 15–31). These statistics are not very different from those for the entire sample, and suggest two rather different interpretations. First, there may be considerably more rape or pressured sex than is directly reported by the teens. Remember that only four teens explicitly said they had been raped. Disclosure of sexual and physical abuse, however, is less likely to be volunteered at the first contact with a young woman. Rather, it tends to be disclosed over time as rapport and trust build. For example, of forty-eight teens who were in the high-risk case-management program with Jorge, six (13%) had disclosed sexual abuse at the time of the ward interview with the TOWs. By the end of a year in the high-risk program, six more, or twelve in all (25%), had confided sexual abuse to Jorge (Erickson and Reyes 1990). Over the years, we also heard many stories of molestation or attempted molestation or sexual abuse of teens by stepfathers, mothers' boyfriends, or other males living in the household. History of sexual abuse has recently been documented in high proportions among teen mothers in several studies (Berenson et al. 1992; Boyer and Fine 1992; Parker et al. 1993).

The second possible interpretation, however, is that culturally, 14- or 15-year-old teens may be considered at a marriageable age. Early union formation might constitute a subcultural pattern. Recall the comments of the young woman from Baja about the young age (by Anglo and Mexican American middle-class standards) by which women expect to become *prometida*. Another Latino cultural institution, the *quinceañera* celebration, occurs when the young woman turns 15, and in Mexico it signals her readiness for courting and marriage (Molina and Aguirre-Molina 1994). It is much like a "coming out" party, celebrated with a Catholic mass and a big party. In form, to an outsider, it looks very much like a wedding, with the young woman and her attendants dressed as bride and bridal attendants, and the young men who escort them dressed in tuxedos. The huge rose garden in Exposition Park in South Central L.A. is a popular site for weddings and picture taking for wedding parties and *quinceañera* parties. I remember during my first years residing in Los Angeles seeing what I now realize were *quinceañera* celebrants there, and wondering why any parent would allow such young girls to be married! Although most of the young girls in this sample would not have had a *quinceañera*, because they are quite expensive, this popular rite of passage may serve as an indication of what may be (or, perhaps, used to be) the appropriate age at transition to adult status in Mexican culture.

In summary, then, the young women tended to have relationships with men who were about five years older than they, who were of similar educational background, and who were members of their same language and ethnic group. The majority of the teens (65%) had a continuing relationship with the baby's father; that is, they were married to, living with, or in a dating relationship to him, but over one-third (35%) stated they had no current relationship with the baby's father. Of the teens who were delivering their second or third child at the interview ($N = 27$, 16%), 77% said their children all had the same father, and 56% were married to or living with him. Although the question of the extent of rape leading to the entry birth in this sample cannot be adequately addressed, it is possible that the actual extent of rape or other forms of sexual abuse, especially among the youngest teens (those under 15 years of age), was higher than that reported to the TOWs.

### Economic Support from Baby's Father

About two-thirds of the young women (63%) thought the baby's father would support them financially, 13% were not sure, and the remaining 25% said he would not (see Table 5.6). Not surprisingly, expectations for economic support were related to the strength of the relationship. Almost all (98%) of those who were married or living together expected economic support from their partners, but only 67% of those who were boyfriend-girlfriend expected support. About one-fifth of the teens in informal relationships or who had no current relationship with the baby's father thought he might provide some economic support, however. This reflects the strong Latino cultural value that men be responsible for the children they father, one of the positive aspects of machismo.

When I asked Blanca and América about this, they indicated that in Mexi-

Table 5.6.      Economic Support Expected from the Baby's Father

|  | Total | | English Speakers | | Spanish Speakers | | U.S. | | Mexico | | Central America | |
|---|---|---|---|---|---|---|---|---|---|---|---|---|
| Variable | N | % | N | % | N | % | N | % | N | % | N | % |
| Will the baby's father support teen and baby? (N = 160)* | | | | | | | | | | | | |
| Yes | 100 | 63 | 40 | 67 | 60 | 60 | 10 | 63 | 63 | 61 | 26 | 63 |
| Not sure | 20 | 13 | 8 | 13 | 12 | 12 | 2 | 12 | 12 | 13 | 6 | 15 |
| No | 40 | 25 | 12 | 20 | 28 | 28 | 4 | 25 | 27 | 26 | 9 | 22 |

* U.S./Mexico: N = 159

can culture it is considered the economic responsibility of the father and/or his family to take care of his offspring. It was their belief, supported by these data, that this ideal is frequently upheld, particularly when the relationship is known in the community. Even married men who father children by other women, a common enough pattern throughout Latin America, are called upon to fulfill their economic obligations to both the first and second family (Pavich 1986, Scrimshaw 1978a).

The rather high level of support and involvement from the baby's father with these young mothers is notable in the context of teenage pregnancy in the United States and has been mentioned by other authors (Becerra and de Anda 1984; Darabi et al. 1986; Erickson 1988). This is in sharp contrast to the situation among African American teen mothers in Baltimore (studied for over a decade by Furstenberg et al. [1987]), for whom there is rarely any long-term involvement or financial support from the baby's father. Another study with African American and white teen mothers showed that only 5% of the fathers of the babies of African American teenage mothers and 39% of those of white teenage mothers under age 18 in Baltimore were married or living with the teen at the time of birth (Hardy et al. 1989). This is quite a bit lower than the proportion found in this sample (53%).

Although we see some evidence of abandonment in this population (3% indicated this explicitly, and another 12% did not elaborate on why there was no relationship), it seems more the exception than the rule. It is also possible that some of the more recently arrived teens were raped on their journey north (Conover 1987), were sent to relatives in the United States to avoid the scandal of an out-of-wedlock birth in Mexico (recall that 11% indicated that the baby's father was not in this country), or came to the United States to deliver the child so the baby would be an American citizen. Since a rather high proportion (29%) of the young mothers had been in the United States for nine months or less when they delivered, these interpretations are certainly plausible. With the tightening of restrictions on immigration policies, delivering a child in the United States may be seen as a viable way to establish a claim to legal residence for the family.

Of the partners who were willing to support their families, 73% were working at the time of the postpartum interview, and another 17% were looking for work. Of those who were working, the majority (58%) were laborers; 17% were transport workers or operatives; and 11% were service workers. It is also probable that some of the partners of the teen mothers were involved in illegal activities such as drug dealing, theft or other criminal behaviors, and the exchange of sex for money (i.e., homosexual prostitution). Such occupations were never revealed in the context of the interview on the postpartum ward, but rather during a subsequent clinic visit, usually in the context of STI (sexually transmitted infection) counseling or risk assessment.[8] For example, Cristina feared that her boyfriend, an illegal immigrant, was prostituting himself in order to make ends meet, and she was afraid of becoming infected with HIV. Several teens had partners who were HIV-positive, having been infected through intravenous drug use. These men were also dealing drugs. Other risk-assessment questions inquired about time spent in jail or gang involvement by either the teen or her partner. Most of the risk of HIV infection incurred by these young women was due to the behavior of their partners (Erickson 1990).

### Social Support

#### Living Arrangements

The young women were asked specifically with whom they were living and the number of adults and children in their household. At the time of the birth most of the teens lived with other adults and children. Only two teens said they lived alone. The mean number of adults in the household was 3.07 ($s = 1.71$, range 1–10) and the mean number of children was 2.55 ($s = 1.5$, range 1–7), for an average household size of 6.62 counting the young mother herself. Most of the teens indicated that they lived in an apartment (60%) rather than a house (39%) or had some other (2%) arrangement.

Of those who said they lived with the baby's father, 83% also lived with other people. Over one-third (37%) lived with his family (17%) or his relatives (20%); 37% with her family (28%) or relatives (9%); and 2% lived with friends or had some other arrangement (7%). Only 17% lived alone with the baby's father.

Of those who did not live with the baby's father, 75% lived with their own family (66%) or relatives (9%), and only 4% lived with his family or relatives. Twelve percent lived with friends, and another 5% had some other arrangement.

Thus, most of these new mothers were living in an extended-family situation and benefited from the economic support of older family members and also from the advice and assistance of persons with more experience in childrearing. Economically and emotionally, at least, teen mothers may indeed be better off when they live with their own families of origin or with the baby's father and his family rather than in a nuclear household, because pooling of resources is possible under marginal economic conditions. As we have seen, fewer than one-fifth of these young mothers formed a nuclear household. Low-income residents in Los Angeles have a difficult time finding affordable housing, and overcrowding is common.

### Perceived Social Support

Most of the young mothers (71%) had family or relatives living in the United States (see Table 5.7). Not surprisingly, 97% of the English speakers and all of the U.S.-born teens had family in the United States. Only about half of the Spanish speakers (54%) had family here, however. Among the foreign-born, 70% of Mexican and 62% of Central American teens had some family in the United States. Overall, 60% had their own mothers here, but only 38% had their fathers. The U.S.-born teens had the highest proportion with their own mothers (94%) and fathers (75%) living in the United States, and the Mexican-born teens had the lowest. Forty-seven percent of the Mexican-born teens had their mothers in the States and 31% had their fathers. Slightly more Central American– than Mexican-born teens had mothers (56%) and fathers (40%) living in the United States, reflecting the different immigration patterns of these two groups.

The teen mothers were asked several questions regarding their perception of the social support available to them. They were asked specifically how supportive the baby's father and their own mothers were, and then asked if there were anyone else, a friend or relative, who was also supportive (up to three more elicited). Over half (63%) said the baby's father was supportive, and 63% indicated their own mother was supportive (see Table 5.8). Over half of the sample (54%) named a third person, 17% a fourth, and two teens (1%) a fifth support person. Most of these other supportive people were female relatives, especially sisters, aunts, and grandmothers (47%); friends (19%); their own fathers (14%); and 15% mentioned some other category of relative (cousin, sister-in-law, mother-in-law, etc.). The teens were also asked whether they had someone who could help them with the baby. Over three-quarters (78%) indicated they did, another 13% were not sure, but only 9% said they had no one to help them.

An overall score was constructed to reflect the degree of social support perceived by the teen. The score summed the level of support (very supportive = 5, supportive = 3, neutral = 1, not very supportive = 0) from each

Table 5.7.    Family Living in United States

| Variable | Total N | Total % | English Speakers N | English Speakers % | Spanish Speakers N | Spanish Speakers % | U.S. N | U.S. % | Mexico N | Mexico % | Central America N | Central America % |
|---|---|---|---|---|---|---|---|---|---|---|---|---|
| Family in U.S. (N = 165)* | 117 | 71 | 62 | 97 | 55 | 54 | 17 | 100 | 73 | 70 | 26 | 62 |
| Mother in U.S. (N = 163)† | 97 | 60 | 57 | 91 | 46 | 40 | 16 | 94 | 58 | 47 | 23 | 56 |
| Father in U.S. (N = 152)‡ | 57 | 38 | 35 | 60 | 22 | 23 | 12 | 75 | 31 | 31 | 14 | 40 |

* U.S./Mexico: N = 164
† U.S./Mexico: N = 163
‡ U.S./Mexico: N = 152


Table 5.8.    Perceived Social Support and Score

| Variable | Total N | Total % | English Speakers N | English Speakers % | Spanish Speakers N | Spanish Speakers % | U.S. N | U.S. % | Mexico N | Mexico % | Central America N | Central America % |
|---|---|---|---|---|---|---|---|---|---|---|---|---|
| Perceived Social Support | | | | | | | | | | | | |
| Baby's Father (N = 173)* | 109 | 63 | 45 | 68 | 64 | 60 | 13 | 66 | 67 | 70 | 28 | 65 |
| Her Mother (N = 173)* | 109 | 63 | 49 | 74 | 60 | 56 | 12 | 71 | 69 | 62 | 27 | 63 |
| Someone to Help (N = 165)† | 128 | 78 | 52 | 83 | 76 | 75 | 10 | 63 | 88 | 83 | 29 | 69 |
| Social Support Score (Possible Range 0–28) (N = 165)† | | | | | | | | | | | | |
| Mean | 10.26 | | 11.46 | | 9.52 | | 12.19 | | 10.02 | | 10.19 | |
| s | 4.48 | | 4.48 | | 4.33 | | 4.09 | | 4.54 | | 4.42 | |
| Range | 0–23 | | 4–23 | | 0–19 | | 5–21 | | 0–23 | | 2–23 | |

s = standard deviation
* U.S./Mexico: N = 172
† U.S./Mexico: N = 165


person named (baby's father, own mother, and up to three others) and whether the teen thought she had someone who could help her with the baby (yes = 3, not sure = 1, no = 0). The higher the score, the greater the level of perceived social support (see Table 5.8).

Only 13% of the teens had a score of five or below, indicating a very low level of perceived social support. The English speakers had a significantly higher social-support score than the Spanish speakers ($t$ = -2.7386, $df$ = 128, $p < .01$), probably reflecting the greater likelihood of their having family living in the United States. This is also reflected in the scores of the U.S.-born teens, whose mean score of 12 was higher than either the Mexican-born teens or the Central American teens, whose mean scores of 10 were the same.

Thus, overall, the majority of these young women perceive that they have a great deal of support from significant others in their lives. Social support has been implicated as an important variable in use of prenatal care and in birth outcome (Boone 1988; Zambrana et al. 1991); thus, it is of considerable interest in the study of Latino teenage pregnancy.

### Risk Status at Postpartum

The TOWs developed a system to "flag" high-risk teens for referral to the high-risk case manager during the time he was still with the Teen Project. The risk factors selected were thought to be possible contributors to less effective contraceptive use, and hence, to repeat pregnancy. There were eight factors that signaled automatic referral to the high-risk case manager: (1) under age 15; (2) multiple birth or multiparous teen; (3) medical complication of teen; (4) medical complication of infant; (5) physical or sexual abuse of teen; (6) substance abuse by teen, her partner, or a family member; (7) severe poverty; and (8) being homeless.

Almost half of the teens (45%) in this sample were identified at risk for one or more of these variables at entry into the program (see Table 5.9). Of these, 85% had one risk, 13% had two identified risks, and 3% had three of these risk factors. Although there were no significant differences among groups, English speakers had a higher proportion under 15 years of age (18%) than Spanish speakers (8%), and the Mexican-born had a higher proportion both under age 15 and with higher parity than U.S.- or Central American–born teens. Other than this, the patterning of risk variables within groups was quite similar. It must be remembered, however, that these risk factors were either self-evident or revealed in an interview shortly after giving birth, before rapport was built with the TOWs. Thus, the prevalence of some of these risk factors may be underestimated, especially those that are more stigmatized (e.g., physical or sexual abuse, drug or alcohol use).

It is the perception of the TOWs that the U.S.-born teens are more likely to be *chola* types, gang and drug involved and part of the inner-city core poverty group. Although this group is the smallest numerically, it is the most difficult with which to work. Middle- and lower-middle-class Mexican Americans move out of East L.A. once their financial resources permit. As Blanca explains, "Once you get a little bit of money, you move to Alhambra.

Table 5.9.    Percentage of Group with Risk Factors at Entry into Teen Project

| | Total N = 173* | | English Speakers N = 66 | | Spanish Speakers N = 107 | | U.S. N = 17 | | Mexico N = 112 | | Central America N = 43 | |
|---|---|---|---|---|---|---|---|---|---|---|---|---|
| | N | % | N | % | N | % | N | % | N | % | N | % |
| None | 95 | 55 | 34 | 52 | 61 | 57 | 12 | 71 | 56 | 60 | 26 | 60 |
| < 15 | 21 | 12 | 12 | 18 | 9 | 8 | 0 | 0 | 17 | 15 | 4 | 9 |
| > para 1 | 26 | 15 | 10 | 15 | 16 | 15 | 2 | 12 | 21 | 19 | 3 | 7 |
| Medical problem | % | | % | | % | | % | | % | | % | |
| Teen | 9 | | 1 | | 7 | | — | | 5 | | 4 | |
| Baby | 5 | | 1 | | 3 | | — | | 3 | | 2 | |
| Substance Use | 5 | | 3 | | 2 | | 1 | | 2 | | 2 | |
| Abuse | 5 | | 2 | | 3 | | 1 | | 0 | | 4 | |
| Poverty | 2 | | 0 | | 2 | | 0 | | 1 | | 1 | |
| Homeless | 1 | | 1 | | 0 | | 0 | | 1 | | 0 | |

*U.S./Mexico: N=172

Nobody wants to stay in East L.A. if they can get out. It's just too rough there."

Even those teens who live in the area do not want to deliver at Women's Hospital. As Jorge notes, "The County is the last resort. You don't want to be seen there. It means you're really poor and you can't go anywhere else." Blanca reinforces this: "The Mexican American girls deliver at White Memorial [a private hospital about half a mile away] or someplace else." Thus, the U.S.-born teens who deliver at Women's Hospital are among the most deprived members of American society.

### Future Plans

At the end of the interview on the postpartum ward, the TOW always asked the young mother what her plans and goals were for the future. The purpose of the question was twofold: first to help the TOW regarding appropriate referrals, and second to encourage the teen to think beyond the present. The question was open ended, and the TOW simply asked the teen what she wanted to do with her life after the postpartum period (four to six weeks after the birth). The goals of the young women are instructive because, for the most part, they are related to school and work rather than domestic life (see Table 5.10). Only a small proportion (11%) of these young women indicate their primary goal is to be a housewife/mother. Many more want to finish high school (47%) and work (24%). Among the groups, the U.S.-born teens are more likely to have high school graduation as a goal (65%) than

Table 5.10.     Percentage of Teens with Selected Plans and Goals for the Future

|  | Total $N = 163†$ | English Speakers $N = 62$ | Spanish Speakers $N = 101$ | U.S. $N = 16$ | Mexico $N = 105$ | Central America $N = 41$ |
|---|---|---|---|---|---|---|
| High school | 47 | 75 | 35 | 69 | 15 | 51 |
| Vocational | 10 | 16 | 9 | 6 | 42 | 17 |
| GED* | 1 | 3 | 0 | 6 | 1 | — |
| College | 1 | 2 | — | 6 | — | 0 |
| Work | 23 | 19 | 24 | 13 | 9 | 27 |
| Housewife | 6 | 8 | 13 | 6 | 23 | 15 |
| Go back home | 4 | 0 | 6 | — | 6 | 0 |

*Certificate of General Educational Development
†U.S./Mexico: N=162

either Mexican-born teens (14%) or Central American–born teens (21%). The only teen mother who said college was her goal was a U.S.-born Latina.

### Perceptions of Women's Roles

A follow-up study in the summer of 1992 explored Latina teen mothers' perceptions of women's roles. Twenty-seven teen mothers, seventeen English speakers and ten Spanish speakers, free-sorted eight roles: Mother, Wife, Housewife, Lover, Girlfriend, Student, Single, and Worker. Each role name was written on a small card in English and Spanish, and the young women arranged these cards into groups based on how they thought the roles seemed to fit together (Bernard 1994). These pile-sort data were analyzed using the multidimensional scaling option in the software package ANTHROPAC (Borgatti 1992; Shelley 1993).[9] Multidimensional scaling is a mathematical tool that provides a visual representation of how conceptually close or far data items are from each other based on respondents' sortings or rankings, which are converted into numerical measures of distance between them (see Kruskal and Wish 1978). Items that are perceived to be more similar to each other will be closer together, and items that are less similar will be farther apart in the visual display. The actual placement of the events on the map means little. It is the distance between events that is important for interpretation.

The resulting multidimensional scaling plot (see Figure 5.1) suggests a clear conceptual distinction between the "homemaker complex," in which Housewife, Wife, and Mother formed a tight group, and the "student complex," in which Student, Single, and Girlfriend were tightly grouped. The two complexes were also perceived to be very different from each other conceptually, as indicated by the distance between them on the multidimen-

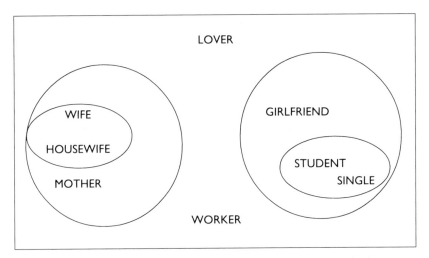

Figure 5.1.    Two-dimensional multidimensional scaling plot of teens' free sort of women's roles
N = 27. Stress = 0.005 after 50 iterations

sional scaling plot. Both Worker and Lover appeared to be conceptually closer to the housewife/mother complex than to the student complex.

The labels the teens gave to the pile groupings also illuminate the meaning they attached to the various roles. For example, Vera, a 17-year-old, single, bilingual Mexican American mother of one who was planning to marry her boyfriend, labeled her pile consisting of Student, Worker, Girlfriend, Lover as "being happy" and her other pile consisting of Mother, Housewife, Wife as "a lot of responsibility." Evelyn, a 17-year-old Central American teen, gave the label *"buena mujer"* (a good woman) to her pile consisting of Mother, Housewife, and Wife. Sonia, a bilingual Mexican mother of two, labeled Student, Worker, and Mother as "most important." Marisa, a single, bilingual mother of one, said that Mother, Wife, Housewife, and Lover constituted "being married" and Student, Worker, Girlfriend, and Single "being single," while Veronica, a U.S.-born teen, labeled the same groups "stuck" and "opportunity." Finally, Ana, a 14-year-old Central American mother of one who lives with her boyfriend, simply said that Mother, Wife, and Housewife were "what I want to be," while Student and Worker were "good" but not what she wanted to be.

The role of Lover (*amante* in Spanish) was difficult for all of the teens to place because, as they indicated, it was thought to be an inappropriate role for Latina women, since it called to mind the image of the "other woman" or the "bad woman" (see the discussion of gender roles in Chapter 2). As the teens were sorting the eight items, Lover was always the last to be placed, and these opportunities were used to explore the meaning of the role to the respondent. For most, it had a strong negative association, but when asked if it could not also be applied to a woman's relationship with her husband or boyfriend, most said yes, but were still somewhat uncomfortable with the term in that respect. Many of the teens left this card in a pile of its own or else qualified it as being the husband's lover and placed it with the home-maker complex. Thus, being your husband's lover was more acceptable than being either your boyfriend's lover or, worst of all, the "other woman." When asked if there were any word in English or Spanish that would convey the sense of being the husband's lover, the teens could not think of any. This pattern held true for both the English and Spanish speakers who partici-pated, although the English speakers seemed to be somewhat more comfort-able with the theme, particularly in its more acceptable format as the hus-band's lover. Traditional gender-role norms still seem to be characteristic of these Latina teen mothers and do not appear to be much affected by accul-turation level.

The teens were also asked to place the eight items in the order of the importance of the role to them, with the first being the most important (as-signed a value of 1) and the last the least important (assigned a value of 8). The ranking exercise suggested that the most important roles for these teens were Student, Mother, and Worker; followed by Wife and Housewife; then Single, Girlfriend, and Lover in that order (see Table 5.11).

The mean ranks for each role reveal that Student was perceived to be the most important role overall and especially for English speakers. Thirty percent ranked it number one in importance. Over half (59%) of the 27 teens ranked it first or second. Overall, Mother was second and Worker third but the top three were ranked differently by English and Spanish speak-ers. Among the Spanish speakers, Mother was ranked first, Student sec-ond, and Worker third. The English speakers ranked Student first, Mother second, and Worker third. Among both English and Spanish speakers the modal rank for both Mother and Student was one. It is important to note here, however, that Mother and Student ranked sixth or seventh in im-portance for almost one-third of the follow-up study sample. Worker had a high ranking because half of the sample (48%) ranked it among the top three.

Wife and Housewife were grouped in the middle range of importance to these young women, but Wife ranked among the top two for about one-third of both English and Spanish speakers. Girlfriend, Single, and Lover ranked as least important, although a small group (about 17%) ranked both Single and Lover among the top two in importance. In contrast, Girlfriend was never ranked better than third.

Table 5.11.      Mean Ranking of Roles

| Role | English Speakers (N = 17) | | | Spanish Speakers (N = 10) | | | Total (N = 27) | | |
|---|---|---|---|---|---|---|---|---|---|
| | Mean | Median | Mode | Mean | Median | Mode | Mean | Median | Mode |
| Student | 2.71 | 2 | 1 | 3.00 | 3 | 1 | 2.82 | 2 | 1 |
| Mother | 3.24 | 2 | 1 | 2.86 | 2.5 | 1 | 3.07 | 2 | 1 |
| Worker | 3.29 | 3 | 2 | 4.20 | 4 | 3 | 3.63 | 4 | 3 |
| Wife | 4.12 | 5 | 5 | 4.40 | 4 | 2 | 4.22 | 5 | 5 |
| Housewife | 4.59 | 4 | 3 | 4.10 | 4.5 | 6 | 4.41 | 4 | 3 |
| Single | 5.53 | 6 | 7 | 4.20 | 4 | 2 | 5.04 | 6 | 7 |
| Girlfriend | 6.35 | 7 | 8 | 7.40 | 8 | 8 | 6.74 | 8 | 8 |
| Lover | 6.18 | 7 | 8 | 5.90 | 6.5 | 7 | 6.07 | 7 | 7 |

These pile-sort results suggest that the stereotype of wife/mother as the most important role for Latina women may be less salient among these young mothers than one would expect from the literature on Latino gender-role values. Overall, these young women, especially the English speakers, seemed to perceive Student, Worker, and Mother as their most important roles, although Worker appears to be less important to the Spanish speakers than to the English speakers.

The pile-sort data support the division between the homemaker and student roles suggested in the comments of teens about the difficulties of going back to school. However, in the ranking of the roles, Student was highest in importance, followed by Mother and then Worker. This suggests that the young mothers do, indeed, recognize the importance of school and work in their lives and futures but also perceive the possible role incompatibility and physical difficulty of being the mother of a young child, and perhaps also a wife, and also being a student or worker or, indeed, all four.

These data suggest that, overall, the Latina teen mothers see finishing school as an important goal and view work as important, perhaps necessary, as well. The mother/wife complex is salient in the multidimensional scaling analysis and among Spanish speakers in the ranking of roles. While most teens ranked Mother high, Wife and Housewife were ranked in the middle. The multidimensional scaling picture may reflect the existing social roles as perceived by the teens, while the ranking may reflect value judgments about the individual roles rather than the way in which they fit together. The high ranking of Student and Worker suggests that the goals of these young women are more in line with middle-class norms than the prior literature suggests. However, they may have difficulty in fulfilling these goals because of the constraints of living in poverty and the additional responsibilities of childrearing.

### Ideal and Real Order of Transition Events

The twenty-seven young women free-sorted ten life events chosen to represent life transitions relevant both to the American cultural script (described in Chapter 2) and to the experience of the teen mothers (see Table 5.12). The education stage (Stage One, high school and college in the American script) was broken down into four transitions (grade school, junior high, high school, and college or university) to account for the fact that most of the young mothers were too young to have completed all the transitions and most had already dropped out of school. Events five and six in the American script (have a boyfriend and live with boyfriend) were included to explore attitudes about where dating or courting behavior fits in the life course. Over one-third of the unmarried teens were actually living with their partners, and recent data on cohabitation in the United States suggest that one-third of women have lived in a cohabiting relationship at some point in their lives (Forrest 1993). Thus, since cohabitation is becoming increasingly common, it seemed important to explore the extent to which this is considered acceptable. Stage Two in the American script is represented by having a job and a career. Marriage and childbearing are the final events studied, representing Stages Three and Four of the American script. The American norms in Table 5.12 represent behavioral norms based on Forrest's (1993) data described in Chapter 2.

The multidimensional scaling map shows a sharp division between the education/career events and the boyfriend/family-formation events (see Figure 5.2). This is reminiscent of the young women's prior division of gender roles into the homemaker and student complexes, often referred to in feminist literature as the private and public spheres of women's lives. The private sphere was separated into two groups: having a boyfriend and living with boyfriend, and marrying and having a baby. The public-sphere events were broken down into three distinct groups: grade school and junior high; high school and university; and career and work.

Some teens referred to having a boyfriend, living with him, getting married, and having a baby as "teenage life," "being serious," "something that has to happen," or "being responsible." This suggests that having a boyfriend is interpreted as being in a serious relationship that is a precursor to marriage and family formation in the minds of many of the young women interviewed. Other teens, however, labeled this constellation of events as something to "avoid while a teen" or as "trouble." Having a baby and getting married, when grouped together without the boyfriend events, were

Table 5.12.        Life Events and Staging of Normative Order for
                   American Script and for Latina Women

| Life Event | American Norm | Latino Norm |
|---|---|---|
| Finish grade school (1 – 6) | 1 | 1 |
| Finish junior high (7 – 9) | 1 | 1 |
| Finish high school (10 – 12) | 1 | 1* |
| Go to college or university | 1 | — |
| Have a boyfriend | — | — |
| Live with boyfriend | 2 | 2 |
| Have a job | 2 | — |
| Have a career | 2 | — |
| Get married | 3 | 4 |
| Have baby/children | 4 | 3 |

* For U.S.-born.

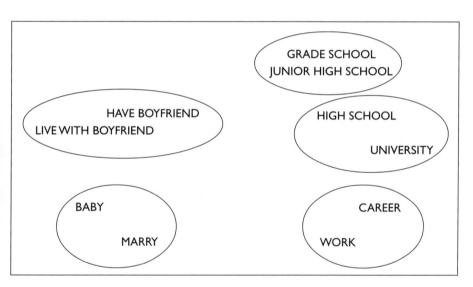

Figure 5.2.    Two-dimensional multidimensional scaling plot of teens' free sort of life events

described as "fulfilling," "*honesta* (honest, virtuous)," and "*una mujer feliz* (a happy woman)."

The teens labeled high school, university, and career as "*estudiante* (student)," "smart, *inteligente* (intelligent)," and "education." Relatively few teens talked about these events as steps in a logical progression toward an end goal over which they had some control, however. Some rather wistfully

Table 5.13.    Ideal and Actual Order of Life Events for Teens and Providers

| Life Event | American Script | Teens' Ideal | Latino Script | Teens' Real |
|---|---|---|---|---|
| Grade school | 1 | 1 | 1 | 1 |
| Junior high | 2 | 2 | 2 | 2 |
| High school | 3 | 3 | 3 | 3 |
| Have boyfriend | 4 | 7 | — | 3 |
| College | 5 | 4 | — | — |
| Work | 6 | 6 | 4 | — |
| Career | 7 | 5 | — | — |
| Marry | 8 | 9 | 6 | — |
| Children | 9 | 10 | 5 | 5 |
| Live with boyfriend* | — | 8 | — | 4 |

* Not applicable for 13 teens and 8 providers.

noted that higher education, work, and career involved having "a future, a good career, or something you wish for," but not, like marriage and family, "something that has to happen." This suggests that the teens are aware of these events as steps to be taken to succeed in middle-class terms, but that they do not always perceive these as necessary or possible in their own lives.

The young women were also asked to sort the events in the order in which they should happen (i.e., the way your parents, teachers, priest, family say they should happen) and the way they actually occurred for them.

Table 5.13 presents the ideal and actual ordinal ranks of the life events for the teens as compared to the American and Latino scripts derived from Forrest's (1993) data. The life event "live with boyfriend" in the ideal script of the teens was ranked by only half of the sample because it was declared inappropriate (i.e., something that should not happen) by 48% of the teens. Thus, more than half of the sample indicated that this was not a normative life event. A similar disagreement over the acceptability of this life event is evident in American society and probably reflects ambivalent views about premarital sexual experience. The respondents who did rank this event placed it close to marriage, indicating the increasingly common practice of cohabitation. Having a boyfriend was arbitrarily assigned a rank of four, to come after the school events, in the American script, although there was no empirical basis for placing it in this position.

For ideal behavior, there was close agreement with the American script about the beginning and ending life events. The teens followed the American script on the first tier of events, which represents primary and secondary schooling. They were also in agreement that the final events should be getting married and having a baby. There was considerable variation in the

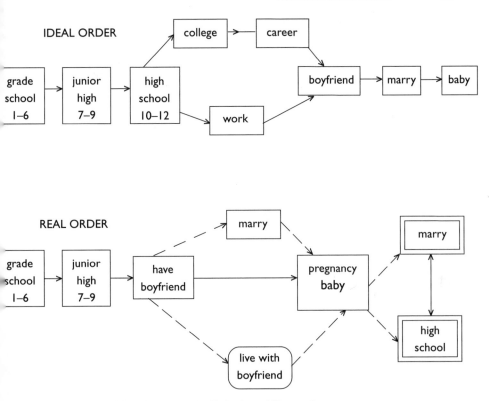

Figure 5.3.     Schematic contrast of the ideal and actual life events for teens

middle events (having a boyfriend, work, college, and career), however. Having a boyfriend was placed immediately before marrying and having a baby. The order of the college, work, and career events was after secondary schooling but before having a boyfriend and family-formation events. The ideal placement of having a boyfriend at the latter end of the process close to marriage suggests that these young women view having a boyfriend as a serious event that leads to family formation. Thus, it appears that the ideal cultural script for these teens is similar to the American middle-class script.

    In fact, the real order of these events in their lives is much more similar to the Latino pattern outlined in Table 5.12 and to the pattern for women below 200% of poverty described earlier (see Table 2.1, Chapter 2). Figure 5.3 provides a schematic contrast of the ideal and actual life events for the teens who participated in this exercise. For the teens, having a boyfriend out of time with their ideal script seemed to thrust them into family formation, bypassing, at least for the time being, high school, the middle career events, and marriage. In this script, one completes school (median ninth grade for Latinos), gets pregnant, lives with a partner, has a baby, and gets married several years after the first birth, suggesting that as with African American adolescents described by Burton (1990), there is an alternative script being played out by low-income Latina teens in East L.A. Unlike the African American teens in Burton's study who allow their own mothers to raise their babies, the Latina teens take on the maternal role and most enter into unions with the baby's father. That the young women recognize the discrepancy between the ideal and the real scripts in their community is summed up by Erica's comment: "You want me to put them in order how it should be or how I see it around here?"

That education and career preparation are truncated by family responsibilities is supported by the future goals of the 173 teen mothers, among whom only 43% wanted to complete high school, less than half thought their chance of doing so likely, and only 1% wanted to go to college. The key event appears to be having a boyfriend early. Strong cultural traditions favoring premarital chastity, female monogamy and fidelity, and traditional gender roles would reinforce the path toward marriage and family formation once sexual intimacy occurred, thus truncating education and the middle-life events among young Latina women. It is probable that "having a boyfriend" is perceived by these Latina teens the way "having a fiancé" used to be perceived in American middle-class culture: as a relationship in which premarital sex often occurred and one that led to marriage and family formation. Indeed, in 1993, exploration of attitudes toward sexual behavior indicated that vaginal intercourse was perceived by almost all participants to be appropriate only between those who are engaged or married (Erickson 1994b). To do otherwise would be to put oneself into the category of "bad woman" or the *amante*. Once a young woman has sex with her boyfriend, she perceives him as her "husband."

In Chapter 2, I made a strong case for the importance of normative life scripts in shaping individual behavior. In order to understand factors that lead to early family formation among Latina adolescents, we must begin to pay more attention to the context and meaning surrounding critical transition events like having a boyfriend, the meaning of school, and the individual teen's perception of the likelihood that she can control the events in her own life. The information presented in this chapter suggests that Latina teen mothers share, at minimum, the ideal of completing high school before getting married and having children, but that they were not able to achieve this ideal in their own lives. Further in-depth study of the cultural meaning of romantic and sexual relationships may further our understanding of factors that must be considered in the prevention of adolescent pregnancy among young Latina teens.

## Summary

It is apparent that in this sample of 173 teen mothers there is wide variety in the actual life circumstances in which the individual teen found herself when she became pregnant. What the young women have in common is that they became mothers before their eighteenth birthday, they are all Latinas, and they delivered in a public hospital in Los Angeles. Beyond this, there are many differences but also some underlying themes.

The young mothers were different in that the English speakers and the U.S.-born were more likely than the Spanish speakers and the foreign-born to be in school when they became pregnant, to have completed a higher education level, and to have higher educational aspirations for the future. In addition, they were less likely to have planned their pregnancies and less likely to be living with their baby's father than were Spanish-speaking and foreign-born teens. In this respect, they conform more to the American pattern of teenage pregnancy as an unplanned event that disrupts schooling.

The teen mothers in the different language and cultural groups were similar, however, with respect to the proportions having some kind of relationship with the baby's father expectations of economic support from him. They were also similar in that most of them had a significant amount of perceived social support. This suggests that, once they become pregnant, all these young women have a similarity of experience as Latinas in L.A. They seem to have a high level of orientation toward family, motherhood, and Latino culture regardless of language preference or country of birth. This was also noted by Scrimshaw et al. (1987) and subsequently by Erickson (1988) during a prior study of birth among Mexican-origin women in L.A. Thus, differences among the teens tend to stem more from actual social and economic circumstances—such as relationship to the baby's father, gender-role orientation, and the social and economic support available to them—than from differences in level of acculturation or culture-group affiliation (i.e., country of birth). While they are not homogenous culturally, there is strong evidence of an overall Latino cultural orientation dominated by strong identification with the maternal role and strong family and partner support networks. Although education was perceived as important, the maternal role took precedence even among the English speakers and U.S.-born who were better schooled and had higher educational aspirations than the Spanish speakers and the foreign-born.

Finally, exploration of life-course norms suggests that the Latino ideal is quite similar to middle-class American norms. However, the actual life course followed by these young women varies considerably from their own ideal and more closely resembles childbearing patterns among poor women in the United States. Cultural values regarding women's roles and sexual behavior reinforce the early childbearing trajectory of these young women. The initiation of sexual intercourse with the boyfriend seems to be equated with long-term commitment to him, especially if pregnancy results. The predominant message young Latinas still receive is that they should be virgins until they marry and should be faithful to their husbands. These cultural messages lead to nonuse of contraception and unintended pregnancy when the teen engages in intercourse. In fact, the teens frequently referred to sexual intercourse as something they could not control in the heat of love and passion, yet were unable to enjoy because of fear and guilt. Pregnancy, motherhood, and marriage or living with the baby's father restore them to the category of "good woman" in which they are rewarded by the support of family and community.

## CHAPTER SIX

# Prenatal Care
# and Birth Outcome

The benefits of prenatal care in reducing maternal and fetal mortality and morbidity are well known, especially in the prevention of low birth weight (less than 2500 grams) in infants. Overall, women who receive no prenatal care are three times more likely to deliver low birth weight infants than women who receive adequate care (Singh et al. 1985), and babies born without the benefit of prenatal care are five times more likely to die in their first year of life (Lazarus and West 1987). Thus, prenatal care has a high cost-benefit ratio, and raising the proportion of women who have adequate prenatal care has been a maternal and child health priority in the United States, especially in the last decade. It is seen as a key factor in reducing the rate of low birth weight, a major contributor to morbidity and mortality among American infants.

The use of prenatal care by teenagers and poor women is notoriously inadequate and has been studied extensively during the past two decades. The Institute of Medicine's (IOM) report on the reasons for underuse of prenatal care implicate a complicated web of impediments including a wide range of physical, psychological, cultural, and economic barriers (Brown 1988). High on the IOM's list are economic barriers that result in lack of access to prenatal care: lack of health insurance, transportation difficulties, shortage of providers who accept Medicaid, and lack of child care for other children. In addition to these economic barriers, lack of knowledge about the importance of prenatal care and its demonstrated efficacy in preventing problems or complications during gestation and delivery (e.g., low birth weight, control of hypertension, diabetes), in combination with a belief that pregnancy and childbirth are normal life events rather than "illnesses," exacerbate underuse or late use of prenatal care services. Another factor that is particularly salient for teenagers is that pregnancy may be unplanned and denied, resulting in nonuse or delayed use of prenatal care.

The TOWs abstracted information regarding prenatal care and labor and delivery outcomes (number of visits, type of delivery, birth weight, complications, etc.) from the medical records of the teen mothers. In addition, teens who had not used prenatal care or had begun prenatal care after the first trimester were asked why they had not gone for care sooner. The questions regarding inadequate prenatal care were open ended, allowing teens to provide their own accounts of their difficulties in trying to get care and reasons they did not go for care. Unfortunately, we did not pursue the use of non-biomedical practitioners in this study, and all the information on prenatal care refers to care within the biomedical health care system in the United States. Fourteen percent of the teens had received prenatal care outside the United States.

Adequate prenatal care is defined as care begun in the first trimester of pregnancy, with at least eight prenatal visits for an uncomplicated pregnancy. The woman is usually seen every four weeks for the first twenty-eight weeks of pregnancy, then every two weeks until the thirty-sixth week, and once a week thereafter until delivery (Andolsek 1990). Normal care includes assessment of overall health, charting of weight gain during gestation, urinalysis, blood pressure and hematocrit screening, and measurement of the growth of the fetus and its position in the womb. With these periodic assessments, health practitioners can monitor the health of the mother and the fetus and identify emergent problems.

Inadequate care, then, includes care begun late (i.e., during the second or third trimester) and fewer than the requisite number of visits per gestational age at time of entry into care. No prenatal care is also inadequate care. It usually indicates that the pregnant woman did not receive any medical care during her pregnancy, although it may also include women who sought care from traditional healers or lay midwives.

Almost a third of the young mothers (30%) had received no prenatal care at all, and another 12% initiated care in the third trimester (see Table 6.1). Thus, 42% of these young mothers had grossly inadequate prenatal care. Only one-fifth of the young women (26%) received care during the first trimester, and only 33% had eight or more prenatal visits. The national rate for Latina women receiving third-trimester or no prenatal care is 12% vs. 9% for African Americans and 4% for non-Latina whites (Singh et al. 1985). Comparable figures for California were 13% for Mexican-born women and 7% for U.S.-born Latina women, compared to 7% for African American women and 4% for non-Latina white women (Williams et al. 1986).

A variable summarizing adequacy of prenatal care was constructed, taking into consideration trimester of entry into care and number of visits (see

Table 6.1.          Adequacy of Prenatal Care (Percentage)

|  | Total | English Speakers | Spanish Speakers | U.S. | Mexico | Central America |
|---|---|---|---|---|---|---|
| | | All (*N* = 171) | | | | |
| *Trimester during which care was initiated:* | | | | | | |
| First | 26 | 24 | 28 | 41 | 22 | 30 |
| Second | 32 | 42 | 25 | 35 | 29 | 37 |
| Third | 12 | 8 | 14 | 6 | 13 | 12 |
| No care | 30 | 26 | 33 | 18 | 36 | 21 |
| Adequate care | 13 | 12 | 13 | 18 | 12 | 14 |
| | | Among Those Receiving Prenatal Care (*N* = 119) | | | | |
| *Trimester during which care was initiated:* | | | | | | |
| First | 38 | 33 | 41 | 50 | 34 | 38 |
| Second | 45 | 57 | 37 | 43 | 46 | 47 |
| Third | 17 | 10 | 21 | 7 | 20 | 15 |
| Adequate care | 19 | 16 | 20 | 21 | 19 | 18 |
| *Number of visits:* | | | | | | |
| < 8 | 67 | 70 | 61 | 53 | 68 | 70 |
| = > 8 | 33 | 30 | 39 | 47 | 32 | 30 |
| Mean | 6.4 | 7.0 | 5.9 | 6.1 | 6.4 | 6.4 |
| *s* | 3.9 | 4.6 | 3.4 | 3.0 | 4.0 | 4.4 |
| Range | 1−24 | 1−24 | 1−20 | 1−10 | 1−20 | 1−24 |

*s* = standard deviation

Table 6.1). It is important to note here that this variable only addresses quantity and timeliness of prenatal care received, not the quality of that care. Adequate care was defined as care begun in the first trimester and eight or more total visits (Andolsek 1990; Kotelchuck 1994). Inadequate care included teens who had some prenatal care but either had not begun care during the first trimester or had fewer than eight visits if care was begun in the first trimester. No care is, by definition, inadequate. By this definition, only 13% of the teens in this sample had adequate prenatal care.

## Acculturation, Country of Origin, and Prenatal Care

There were virtually no differences between English and Spanish speakers regarding adequacy of prenatal care. Although there was a tendency for Spanish speakers to have a greater proportion receiving no prenatal care at all, this did not reach statistical significance. Among the cultural groups, the U.S.-born teens tended to receive more adequate care than the foreign-born teens, especially care beginning during the first trimester of pregnancy. Once again, however, the trend did not reach statistical significance.

Among the teens who went for prenatal care, 38% had their first visit during the first trimester, 45% in the second trimester, and the remaining 17% in the last trimester. Similar data for California suggest that Mexican-born women had the lowest proportion beginning prenatal care during the first trimester (59%) compared to 71% for U.S.-born Latinas, 73% for African American women, and 82% for non-Latina white women (Williams et al. 1986).

The mean number of prenatal visits among those who had received care was 6.4 and ranged from 1 to 24. Thus, among teens who received care, only 19% received adequate care. By all measures, then, the young women in this study had received inadequate prenatal care and were much worse off than women at both state and national levels.

## Source of Prenatal Care

There is a range of health care providers in Los Angeles County who provide obstetric and gynecological services to women, including both public and private providers. The county health care system is comprised of a system of public clinics and sub-centers and is probably the largest provider of reproductive health care for poor Latina women in L.A. At the time of the study, all poor, pregnant women were eligible for Medi-Cal coverage for pregnancy, labor, and delivery if they met the income eligibility requirements, regardless of their legal status in the United States. All of the county clinics accepted Medi-Cal reimbursement, but this varied among the private clinics.

There were thirty-three health centers in the county, twenty-eight of which provided prenatal care services during the time of the study (see Table 6.2). These health centers funneled women into the four county hospitals (LAC-USC Women's Hospital, Martin Luther King Hospital-UCLA, Harbor General Hospital-UCLA, and Olive View Hospital-UCLA) for labor and delivery. Women's Hospital received labor and delivery patients primarily from the East and Metro-West County Health Centers, which are geographically closest to the hospital, but it also received high-risk cases from throughout the county system.

Among the teens who received prenatal care, the largest provider of that care was the county health system, which accounted for over half (53%) of the prenatal care services provided to the teens (see Table 6.3). It is also probable that some of the teens who received care in the other L.A. clinics and hospitals were also utilizing county services, although the actual names of the sites were not coded.

Table 6.2.    Los Angeles County Health Facilities

| Health Centers | Prenatal Care | Family Planning |
|---|---|---|
| East County Health Centers | | |
| (A) LAC/USC Medical Centers | yes | yes |
| (1) Edward R. Roybal Health Center | yes | yes |
| (2) Northeast Health Center | yes | yes |
| (3) Whittier Health Center | yes | yes |
| (4) Pico Rivera Subcenter | yes | yes |
| San Gabriel Valley County Health Centers | | |
| (5) El Monte Comprehensive Health Center | yes | yes |
| (6) Pomona Health Center | yes | yes |
| (7) La Puente Subcenter | yes | yes |
| (8) Alhambra Health Center | yes | yes |
| (9) Monrovia Health Center | yes | no |
| (10) Azuza Health Center | yes | no |
| Metro-West County Health Centers | | |
| (11) H. Claude Hudson Health Center | yes | yes |
| (12) Hollywood Wilshire Health Center | yes | no |
| (13) West Hollywood Subcenter | STD treatment only | STD treatment only |
| (14) Central Health Center | yes | yes |
| (15) Ruth Temple Health Center | yes | yes |
| (16) Yvonne Burke Health Center | yes | yes |
| (17) Culver City Subcenter | yes | yes |
| (18) Venice Subcenter | yes | yes |
| Metro-South County Health Centers | | |
| (B) King-Drew (MLK)/UCLA Medical Center | yes | yes |
| (19) Hubert H. Humphrey Comprehensive Health Center | yes | yes |
| (20) Compton Health Center | no | no |
| (21) Dollarhide Health Center | yes | yes |
| (22) Paramount Health Center | yes | yes |
| (23) San Antonio Health Center | yes | yes |
| (24) Bell Gardens Subcenter | yes | yes |
| (25) South Health Center | yes | yes |
| (26) Florence/Firestone Subcenter | yes | yes |
| (27) Curtis R. Tucker Health Center | no info. | no info. |
| (28) Imperial Heights Subcenter | yes | yes |
| (29) Lawndale Subcenter | yes | yes |
| Coastal County Health Centers | | |
| (C) Harbor/UCLA Medical Center | yes | yes |
| (30) Long Beach Comprehensive Health Center | no | no |
| (31) Harbor/San Pedro Health Center | yes | yes |
| (32) Wilmington Subcenter | yes | yes |
| (33) Avalon Subcenter | no info. | no info. |

Table 6.3.     Source of Prenatal Care (Percentage)

|  | Total | English Speakers | Spanish Speakers | U.S. | Mexico | Central America |
|---|---|---|---|---|---|---|
|  | N = 115 | N = 48 | N = 65 | N = 12 | N = 68 | N = 32 |
| Source * |  |  |  |  |  |  |
| County clinics | 53 | 48 | 57 | 33 | 53 | 59 |
| Mexico/COB† | 14 | 6 | 20 | 17 | 18 | 6 |
| L.A. hospitals | 11 | 17 | 6 | 8 | 6 | 22 |
| L.A. clinics | 8 | 8 | 8 | 8 | 9 | 6 |
| Other CA | 8 | 8 | 8 | 17 | 7 | 6 |
| Private doctor | 6 | 13 | 2 | 17 | 7 | 0 |

* L.A. hospitals and clinics unspecified
† Country of birth

Among the clinics most commonly used by this sample, accounting for 41% of prenatal care delivered to these teens, were Women's Hospital (13%), Central (14%), Hudson (9%), and Roybal (5%). Another 11% of the teens used another of the clinics listed in Table 6.2. Other hospital clinics (11%) and other clinics in the L.A. basin (8%) accounted for another 19% of prenatal care, and probably many of these were also part of the county system as noted above.

Overall, only 6% of the teens relied on a private physician for prenatal care. In the Latino community there are many private medical doctors (PMDs) and private clinics that can be used on a fee-for-service basis. Some of these accept Medi-Cal and others do not. The English-speaking teens and the U.S.-born teens were the most likely to have utilized a private physician for care.

Fourteen percent of the teens in this sample indicated that they had received prenatal care in Mexico or their country of origin, and another 8% received care in a different part of California or the United States.

### Reasons for Inadequate Care

Teens who had no prenatal care or who did not initiate care during the first trimester of pregnancy were asked why they did not go sooner. The most frequently cited reasons included financial problems (25%), not thinking it was important because she felt fine (15%), problems getting appointments (12%),[1] "just didn't go" (15%). Less frequently mentioned reasons included not knowing where to go (7%); not knowing she was pregnant (4%); fear of the hospital, clinic, or pelvic exam (3%); and time conflicts with school or work (2%).

The reasons given by these teens echo those in the Institute of Medicine's report on the crisis in prenatal care in the United States (Brown 1988). The barriers to care for these teens fall into three major categories: financial, structural, and personal. All three contributed to inadequate prenatal care in this group.

### Social Factors and Adequacy of Care

Because prenatal care has been widely regarded as one of the most important variables in promoting a good birth outcome, it is of interest to explore social variables that might be associated with early and adequate care. In a study of Mexican-origin adolescent primiparas (mothers bearing a first child) in L.A. in 1981–1982, I found that having a planned pregnancy was the only significant variable associated with better prenatal care, although the amount of variation explained was only 6% (Erickson 1988).[2]

Regression analysis was performed using trimester at initiation of prenatal care as the dependent variable and age, social support, U.S./foreign-born, relationship to the baby's father, language preference, and whether the pregnancy was planned as independent variables. Results were not significant. Discriminant analysis was also performed classifying the teens into either adequate or inadequate care using the strict definition defined above. Again, results were inconclusive, with almost 40% misclassification based on these same independent variables. These results suggest that none of these social variables, either separately or in combination, explain adequacy of prenatal care for this sample. The teens' own report of reasons they did not go for care indicate that system factors such as cost, transportation difficulties, and lack of knowledge about where to go and about the importance of prenatal care were more important reasons for inadequate care than were social factors.

### Birth Outcomes

Birth-outcome variables, such as birth weight and complications of labor and delivery, were abstracted from the medical record by the TOWs who reviewed the mothers' labor and delivery charts before they interviewed the teens on the ward. There were 155 labor and delivery records available for review.

### Birth Weight

The mean birth weight for the sample was 3001.6 grams, with a range of 430 to 4400 grams. Almost one-fifth of the teens in this sample (18%) delivered a low birth weight (< 2500 grams) baby, of which 23% were very low birth weight (< 1500 grams). This proportion of low birth weight is about twice that found in a national study of births to Latina teens aged 19 and under (9.3%; Balcazar and Aoyama 1991); more than twice that of Latina teens in California (7%; Brindis and Jeremy 1988); and about twice the rate of teens aged 17 and under surveyed at Women's Hospital in 1986–1987 (8%) and 1992–1994 (9%). These differences are attributable to the fact that this is a high-obstetric-risk population.

The proportion of low birth weight babies was higher among Spanish speakers (21%) than among English speakers (14%), but the difference was not statistically significant. Among the cultural groups, those born in the United States had the lowest proportion of low birth weight babies, 11%, compared to 17% of those born in Mexico and 23% of those born in Central America. All of the very low birth weight babies were born to foreign-born teens. This is an interesting finding because it is the reverse of the trend among all Latina births, in which foreign maternal birth is associated with better birth outcomes. Rates of low birth weight have been shown to be lowest among Mexican-born women, 5.0%, compared to 6.3% among U.S.-born Latinas, 5.7% among whites, and 14.5% among African Americans (Balcazar and Aoyama 1991). California rates repeat this pattern but are even lower: 4% for Mexican-born women, 5% for U.S.-born Latinas, 5% for non-Latina whites, and 11% for African Americans (Williams et al. 1986). There were only seventeen U.S.-born teens in this sample, and it is difficult to draw any definite conclusions based on such a small group, but these results raise the possibility that foreign birth may not confer a protective effect on young Latina teens, especially those from Central America.

### Adequacy of Care and Birth Weight

Regression analysis was performed using baby's birth weight as the dependent variable and age, adequacy of prenatal care, relationship to the baby's father, the social support score, whether the baby was planned, language preference, and country of birth as independent variables. In this regression, adequacy of prenatal care emerged as the only significant variable.[3] The overall regression was significant at probability .10 but explained only 3% of the variation (see Table 6.4). These results suggest that there is a weak positive association between adequacy of prenatal care and birth weight in this sample.

### Infant Complications

One-fifth (23%) of the infants had fetal complications noted in the mother's record. The most common was meconium passage (11%), followed by fetal distress (7%) and prematurity (6%). Thirty-three of the infants (21%)

Table 6.4.    Regression Coefficients of Predictor Variables on Birth Weight ($N = 149$)

| Predictor Variable | Parameter Estimate | Standardized Estimate |
|---|---|---|
| Intercept | 1941.35 | 0.00* |
| Age | 76.52 | 0.12 |
| Prenatal care adequacy | −51.28 | −0.17* |
| Relationship to baby's father | 10.55 | 0.01 |
| Acculturation | 188.96 | 0.14 |
| U.S.-born | 76.04 | 0.03 |
| Pregnancy planned | −26.33 | −0.02 |
| Overall $F$ | 1.79 | |
| Probability $> F$ | 0.10 | |
| Adjusted R-square | 0.03 | |

*significant at .05

had baby complications noted. The major complication was prematurity. Nine percent of the infants were premature (14 babies), three of whom were sent to the Neonatal Intensive Care Unit after birth.

## Maternal Complications

The majority of the teen mothers had no maternal complications (69%). Among the 31% who did, however, the problems were serious. Thirteen percent of all the mothers had hypertensive disorders (i.e., toxemia, eclampsia), 9% amnionitis, 3% a prior medical problem, 1% diabetes, 1% hemorrhage, and the remaining 4% had some other problem.

Fifteen percent of the mothers had obstetric problems, including three teens with multiple gestation, six with malpresentation, three with dysfunctional labor, two with shoulder dystocia, one each with uterine atony and abruptio placenta, and seven with some other problem.

## Type of Delivery

The majority of the young mothers in this sample had a spontaneous vaginal delivery (71%), and another 9% had a vaginal delivery aided by vacuum or forceps. The cesarean section rate in this group was 20%. There were no differences in type of delivery among the different language or culture groups.

## Breast-feeding Plans

One of the educational goals of the Teen Project was to encourage teens to breast-feed. This was incorporated into the project by asking questions about breast-feeding at each contact with the teen mother and by promoting breast-feeding at the postpartum contact. When the young women were interviewed on the postpartum ward, 21% ($N = 33$) said they intended to breast-feed and another 41% ($N = 63$) intended to breast-feed and supplement with bottle-feeding. Over one-third ($N = 57$; 37%), however, did not plan to breast-feed their babies at all. Thus, overall, 62% of the young mothers intended to breast-feed at the time they were interviewed in the hospital, a proportion only slightly lower than that found in studies of Latina women in Southern California, 78% to 82% (Romero-Gwynn and Carias 1989; Scrimshaw et al. 1987).

The English-speaking teens (69%) were more likely than the Spanish-speaking teens (57%) to indicate they were going to breast-feed. Among the cultural groups, the U.S.-born were the most likely of the three groups (82% vs. 61% of Mexican- and 69% of Central American–born teens) to be planning to breast-feed. As with low birth weight, the pattern is opposite that of studies that include adult women, in which the foreign-born and the Spanish-speaking are more likely to breast-feed than the U.S.-born and English-speaking Mexican Americans (John and Martorell 1989; Romero-Gwynn and Carias 1989; Scrimshaw et al. 1987).

Of those intending to breast-feed, by the time of the postpartum appointment four weeks after the birth, 70% indicated they were still breast-feeding. An additional fifteen teens who had indicated in the initial interview that they did not plan to breast-feed were breast-feeding at the time of the postpartum visit, however. Of the teens who came for their postpartum appointment ($N = 141$) and responded to the question on breast-feeding ($N = 120$), less than half (43%), overall, were breast-feeding their infants. Thus, while breast-feeding begins as the preferred infant feeding method, by the time of the postpartum appointment, more than half (55%) of the mothers have already ceased breast-feeding.

In summary, the teens in this sample were an at-risk obstetric population. Thirteen percent of these young mothers had hypertensive disorders, 9% had amnionitis, and 9% had other serious medical problems. Very few, 13%, received truly adequate prenatal care; 44% received intermediate care; and 43% received third-trimester or no care. Lack of access and lack of knowledge, rather than social context variables, were the primary reasons for inadequate care. Birth outcomes reflect this. Almost one-fifth, 18%, had low birth weight babies, and 6% had premature infants. Most, 62%, were planning to breast-feed.

Differences by acculturation and country of birth were apparent. A larger proportion of U.S.-born than foreign-born teens had adequate prenatal care and used private physicians, suggesting, perhaps, that they knew the system better and were better off financially. Birth outcomes and breast-feeding intentions of this high-risk, young maternal population were opposite those found in most studies of Latino births. The U.S.-born teens and English speakers had a lower proportion delivering low birth weight infants and a greater proportion planning to breast-feed than the foreign-born and Spanish speakers. Future studies should investigate generation and acculturation effects on birth outcome among Latina adolescents.

### Case Studies

Five case studies were chosen to illustrate the interaction of social circumstances, use of prenatal care, and birth outcome.

#### *Rosa, raped by mother's boyfriend*

Rosa is a 16-year-old Spanish-speaking teen from El Salvador who has lived in the United States for one year. She lives with her mother, two sisters, and a brother. Rosa was attending high school (tenth grade) when she was raped by her mother's boyfriend, a 28-year-old Guatemalan, who is currently incarcerated for the assault. Rosa became pregnant as a result of the rape, dropped out of school, and delivered a premature (23-week-old), very low birth weight (2 lb. 13 oz.) male infant by cesarean section in December. Rosa only made three prenatal visits during her pregnancy.

The baby had multiple medical problems, including blindness and genetic problems. He was hospitalized for three months and has had to have surgery since being discharged from the hospital in March. Rosa came to the clinic for her postpartum appointment and chose oral contraceptives at that visit. However, she never began taking them and missed several follow-up appointments because she had to take care of her infant. Rosa did not have a sexual partner during her contact with our project and has relied on abstinence for pregnancy prevention. Rosa's case was closed in January, thirteen months after her delivery, because she had no need of the contraceptive services available at the clinic.

#### *Sylvia, planned pregnancy but abandoned by baby's father*

Sylvia, a 15-year-old Spanish-speaking teen from Nicaragua, has been in the United States for three years. In April she delivered a 4 lb. 6 oz. infant with breech presentation by cesarean section. The baby had serious medical complications that required surgery. Sylvia had good prenatal care. She initiated care during the first trimester and had ten prenatal visits. She lives with her mother and four brothers and sisters. Sylvia's father is missing in Nicaragua.

Sylvia was in school when she became pregnant but dropped out after completing ninth grade. She would like to go back to school but needs to help her mother take care of the baby. Sylvia intended to get pregnant, although she said her 19-year-old boyfriend did not want her to have a baby. He left her when he found out she was pregnant and denies he is the father. Sylvia confided to the counselor that she tried to kill herself by taking some pills when she found out she was pregnant, but she never told anyone about it.

Sylvia failed to keep her postpartum appointment several times, primarily because of transportation and child-care difficulties, but finally came in June. She was diagnosed with condyloma (genital warts) and admitted to having multiple sexual partners—more than four in the previous twelve months and more than ten since her sexual debut at age 11. Her last sexual partner had been in and out of jail, was a drug dealer, and was involved in gang activities. He also used alcohol, marijuana, and cocaine. Sylvia has only used alcohol in the past. She chose oral contraceptives but was unable to come to the clinic for subsequent follow-up.

Sylvia needed treatment for condyloma in July, but since her postpartum appointment, follow-up has been difficult. Her phone is often disconnected, and she moved three times between June and September. In October she came to the clinic and received treatment for her condyloma, but she has failed to attend her follow-up appointments. In January she moved again, quite far from our clinic, and her case was closed.

### Gloria, chola *lifestyle*

Gloria, a 16-year-old, English-speaking, U.S.-born teen, began prenatal care at the beginning of the second trimester of pregnancy and had only two prenatal visits because of financial reasons. She and her partner, Juan, a 23-year-old, U.S.-born, bilingual gang member, live with friends. Gloria was not in school when she became pregnant and was "staying at home doing nothing." She used cocaine throughout the first trimester of pregnancy, but stopped when she found out she was pregnant. She delivered a healthy 8 lb. 1 oz. baby girl with no complications. She thinks that the baby is a good reason for her and Juan to start over and "straighten out our lives . . . now we have a chance [the baby]." Nevertheless, Gloria does not think Juan intends to support her and the baby, even though she says they had both wanted the pregnancy. He was spending some time in jail. She intends to go back to school and get her GED and to rely on AFDC, Medi-Cal, and WIC for economic support until she gets a job.

Gloria never came to the clinic for her postpartum appointment and was unable to be contacted by phone or mail.

### Patricia, *unplanned pregnancy*

Patricia is a 17-year-old Mexican American who had dropped out of school at age 16 after tenth grade. She was working as a receptionist at the time she became pregnant by Miguel, an 18-year-old Latino she was dating. Although she knew about birth control, she didn't use anything because she wasn't planning to have sex with Miguel, and they never talked about it. She never told Miguel she was pregnant. Patricia did not go for prenatal care because she was considering having an abortion. She said that she didn't take care of herself because she was going to terminate the pregnancy. She said:

> I used to go out and party and drink and then I found out it was too late to terminate, and I started to care and took vitamins. . . . Two days later I started to cramp and my mother brought me to the hospital and they told me I was in labor. I had the baby and he died the same day. I'm just glad it's all over now.

Patricia's baby, delivered at 25–26 weeks, weighed less than 1100 grams. At one clinic visit, she told her TOW:

> I didn't want my life to be like this. I wanted to get married and have a baby from someone I love. I didn't love this guy. . . . He has another girl pregnant, and she is going through with it. . . . I hate him and don't want to have anything to do with him.

In the year following the baby's death, Patricia "partied" a lot. She had eight sexual partners but was a consistent user of foam and condoms for both pregnancy and STI prevention. Although she never finished high school, she continued to work. At age 18, about two years after she entered the Teen Project, she fell in love, got married, and got pregnant. She and her husband are very happy about the pregnancy, and she began prenatal care right away.

### Perla, a housewife

Perla came to the United States from Mexico less than a year before she gave birth to her son at age 14. Perla was one of the few teens with adequate prenatal care (first trimester, nine visits), and she had no complications with the birth despite her young age. She is living with the baby's father, José, and they plan to marry. He is 19 and has only completed third grade. He works as a cook full-time and helps support the family. They live with his family: seven other adults and two children. The extended family is supportive and happy about the baby, which was a planned and wanted child.

Perla used oral contraceptives for two years following the birth of her son. She was still with the baby's father when she graduated to the adult clinic at age 18. Perla finished sixth grade in Mexico and had expressed a desire to go to school in the United States. However, she never went to school and devotes herself to being a wife and mother. She and José are thinking about having another child.

These case studies illustrate the complex interactions between social context factors, use of prenatal care, birth outcome, and subsequent contraception not captured in the quantitative data. For the three cases with low birth weight infants, two had poor or no prenatal care and the third had good prenatal care. All three, however, had substantial psychosocial stress regarding their partners: rape, abandonment, and indifference.

Rosa had an unplanned pregnancy as a result of a rape, and although she received prenatal care, delivered a very low birth weight infant with multiple medical problems. In fact, Rosa may have subconsciously been trying to provoke a miscarriage, although she never said this. Sylvia was abandoned by her partner when he found out she was pregnant and was so distraught that she tried unsuccessfully to take her own life. Patricia, whose preterm infant died, had an unplanned pregnancy. She hadn't planned on having sex with her boyfriend, whom she now despises. She was going to have an abortion and did not take care of herself until she found out it was too late to terminate.

These cases suggest that the extent to which the pregnancy was wanted and the quality of the relationship to the father of the baby are important factors in the willingness of the woman to take care of herself during pregnancy. Although this was not borne out statistically in this small sample, other studies have shown that the extent to which the pregnancy is wanted is associated with earlier prenatal care (Joyce and Grossman 1990). A woman with an unwanted pregnancy may go for prenatal care, but she may go late, miss appointments, and lack the will to take care of herself beyond that. The nature of the relationship with the partner can sometimes redefine a wanted pregnancy into an unwanted one, as in Sylvia's case, and have an impact on subsequent self-care during the pregnancy as well.

Perla exemplifies the stereotype of the "good mother." She is a recent immigrant from Mexico, Spanish-speaking, and completed only sixth grade. She is living in a stable relationship with a supportive partner who is working. Her pregnancy was planned, and she received good prenatal care. Although she gave birth at a young age, she delivered a healthy infant with no complications.

Gloria started taking care of herself (i.e., stopped using drugs) when she found out she was pregnant but did not receive adequate prenatal care for financial reasons. She perceived the pregnancy as a chance for a new life. She delivered a healthy infant.

Teen mothers' life circumstances also influence postpartum care and contraceptive use. For example, both Rosa and Sylvia, who had low birth weight infants, had difficulty in complying with clinic attendance and contraceptive protocols. Rosa failed to comply with the follow-up regimen for oral contraceptives for two reasons: she found clinic return difficult due to her baby's medical problems, and she did not have a sexual partner and was abstinent. Sylvia's lifestyle subsequent to her baby's birth—multiple sexual partners, STI, a partner involved in drugs and gangs, and transient living arrangements—made it difficult for her to comply with medical treatment for STI and follow-up for contraception. Lack of a stable home, income, and someone to help her care for the baby seem to be the primary impediments to clinical follow-up for Sylvia. Gloria, like so many of the *cholas*, never came for her postpartum appointment and could not be contacted. Perla and Patricia were consistent contraceptors: Perla for child spacing and Patricia for STI and pregnancy prevention until she found "the right guy."

These five cases strongly suggest that the circumstances surrounding the pregnancy and the teen's relationship to the baby's father have a significant influence on her use of prenatal care and self-care during pregnancy. Thus, it is important to address the major reasons for unwanted (15%) and unintended (48%) pregnancy: sexual abuse, instrumental use of pregnancy for other ends (e.g., to get out of a lifestyle incompatible with the maternal role, to fulfill unmet emotional needs, to force commitment from the partner), and lack of contraceptive use (e.g., unplanned sex or denial of possibility of pregnancy).

Because adequacy of prenatal care is associated with better birth outcomes—influencing birth weight even in this small high-risk sample—efforts to improve adequacy of care among Latina teens must address the reasons for late or nonuse of prenatal care given by these young women, namely, lack of access to health care (due to cost, location, or transportation) and lack of knowledge about where to go and about the importance of prenatal care. These are policy issues that can only be addressed at the societal level—in the health care system, in the economic system, and in public education.

Although I have spent a great deal of this chapter dwelling on negative aspects of childbearing in this high-risk group, despite poverty, poor prenatal care, and young maternal age, the majority (over 80%) of these teen mothers delivered healthy infants. Most had either planned (37%) or welcomed (48%) the pregnancy. The majority (65%) had a relationship with the baby's father. Almost all enjoyed the support of their family and friends. More than half were like Perla, married or in stable unions and actively involved in the process of family building. Supported by a culture that values motherhood and family, the majority of these young Latina mothers had overcome tremendous odds against a healthy birth.

## CHAPTER SEVEN

# Prevention of Repeat Pregnancy

The young mothers in the Teen Project were an at-risk obstetric population with significant social, economic, psychological, and medical risk factors. Most could also be considered at risk for rapid repeat pregnancy, since the majority were married, lived with their partner, or were in dating relationships. In addition, the majority were already out of school and likely to remain so postpartum, even though they recognized the value of school and work. Over half spoke only Spanish, further limiting their access to education and employment in the United States. Of these, probably a significant proportion were residing in the United States illegally and are likely to remain part of the growing "underclass" of undocumented, working-poor immigrants in Los Angeles.

The Teen Project itself was a hospital-based program situated in a family planning clinic, which was the high-risk referral clinic for the county health system. Because of hospital rules, all care was clinic based and there was no home visiting, although telephone and mail follow-up was extensively used. Within these constraints, the TOWs tried to provide the most comprehensive services they could and maintained a warm, welcoming ambiance in the teen room. In contrast to regular clinic services, the TOWs took more time with the teens, saw them on a walk-in basis, and rarely turned anyone away no matter how early or late they arrived for an appointment. Thus, many clinic barriers were removed. This extra care and the extensive follow-up (described in Chapter 3) was the intervention. The combination of caring health personnel, attention to the teen's concerns, and intensive follow-up was expected to help facilitate contraceptive use, thereby preventing repeat pregnancy.

How effective was the Teen Project in achieving this goal? Table 7.1 provides information on the one- and two-year follow-up samples for the Hewlett Project. The one-year follow-up group consisted of 173 cases and 100 controls[1] recruited on the postpartum ward between April 1, 1989, and December 30, 1990. The two-year group consisted of 78 cases and 60 controls recruited between April 1 and December 30, 1989, who were eligible for two-year follow-up in December 1991 when the project ended.

The evaluation design compared two outcome measures for cases and controls, assuming that, all other things being equal, better outcomes among the cases would be attributable to the intervention. The outcome measures were (1) retention in family planning care, and (2) repeat pregnancy at one and two years after program entry. Appendix B provides a detailed description of how these variables were measured.

### Contraceptive Knowledge and Use Postpartum

At the time of the interview on the postpartum ward, about half of the teens (49%) said they knew about birth control, and 31% of the young women had talked with their partners about birth control (see Table 7.2). A slightly larger proportion of teens with planned pregnancies (37%) had talked about contraception compared to those who had not been actively seeking pregnancy (28%). A greater proportion of English speakers (38%) than Spanish speakers (26%) said they had discussed contraception with their partner. U.S.-born teens were the most likely of the three cultural groups to have discussed contraception with their partners (38%), followed closely by Mexican-born teens (34%). Central American–born teens were the least likely (20%) to have discussed contraception with their partners. Even though a considerable number knew about birth control, very few of the young mothers, only 13%, had ever used contraception in the past. Significantly more English-speaking (61%) than Spanish-speaking teens (42%) knew about contraception (chi-square $= 5.599$, $df = 1$, $p < .05$), but more of the Spanish speakers had used it in the past (21% of Spanish speakers vs. 7% of English speakers). Thus, the English-speaking teens, overall, were more likely to know about contraception and to have talked with their partners about birth control, but less likely to have used it in the past. Among the cultural groups, the U.S.-born teens, however, were more likely than either group of foreign-born teens to have used contraception in the past. The teen mothers who had previously had a child (multiparous teens) were more likely to know about birth control than those having their first baby (67% vs. 46%, $p < .07$), probably because of prior access to information during postpartum care, but there were no differences in past use of contraception.

Teens who said they knew about birth control ($N = 81$) were asked to name the methods of which they were aware. This was a spontaneous mention of methods by the teen rather than a recognition of methods read by

Table 7.1.    Program Retention for Postpartum Teen Mothers

| | Case | | Control | | Total | |
|---|---|---|---|---|---|---|
| | *N* | % | *N* | % | *N* | % |
| Recruitment Period: One-Year Sample (4/1/ 89 – 12/30/90) | | | | | | |
| Eligible | 173 | 100 | | | 273 | |
| Follow-up | 172 | | 99 | | 268* | |
| Active at one year | 73 | 42 | 13 | 13 | 86 | 32 |
| Lost to follow-up | 99 | 58 | 83 | 87 | 182 | 68 |
| Recruitment Period: Two-Year Sample (4/1/89 – 12/30/89) | | | | | | |
| Eligible | 78 | | 60 | | 138 | |
| Lost in first year | 54 | 69 | 58 | 97 | 112 | 81 |
| Follow-up | 24 | | 2 | | 26† | |
| Active at two years | 16 | 67/21† | 1 | 50/2‡ | 17 | 69/12‡ |
| Lost to follow-up | 8 | 33/10‡ | 1 | 50/2‡ | 9 | 31/3‡ |

*Excludes 5 with unavailable medical records
†Excludes 3 with unavailable medical records
‡First number is percentage of those remaining, second is percentage of those eligible

Table 7.2.    Contraception and Reproductive Plans

| | | | English | Spanish | | | Central |
| | Total | | Speakers | Speakers | U.S. | Mexico | America |
| *Variable* | *N* | % | % | % | % | % | % |
|---|---|---|---|---|---|---|---|
| Know BC* | 164 | 49 | 61 | 42 | 56 | 51 | 42 |
| Ever talk | 160 | 31 | 38 | 26 | 38 | 34 | 20 |
| Used BC | 157 | 13 | 7 | 21 | 25 | 16 | 0 |
| Want BC | 152 | 79 | 77 | 80 | 87 | 81 | 70 |
| More kids | 154 | | | | | | |
| yes | | 19 | 15 | 22 | 25 | 18 | 19 |
| maybe | | 35 | 50 | 25 | 56 | 30 | 40 |
| no | | 46 | 35 | 53 | 19 | 52 | 41 |
| *N* more | 88 | | | | | | |
| Mean | | 1.49 | 1.51 | 1.47 | 1.22 | 1.30 | 2.04 |
| *s* | | 1.19 | 1.52 | 0.86 | 0.44 | 0.57 | 2.08 |
| Range | | 1 – 10 | 1 – 10 | 1 – 5 | 1 – 2 | 1 – 3 | 1 – 10 |
| How soon † | 77 | | | | | | |
| Mean | | 4.38 | 4.75 | 4.05 | 4.11 | 4.49 | 4.18 |
| *s* | | 1.44 | 1.56 | 1.26 | 1.67 | 1.24 | 2.07 |
| Range | | 1 – 10 | 1 – 10 | 2 – 6 | 2 – 5 | 2 – 8 | 1 – 10 |
| Total kids | 127 | | | | | | |
| Mean | | 1.87 | 2.08 | 1.74 | 2.0 | 1.69 | 2.32 |
| *s* | | 1.20 | 1.49 | 0.96 | 0.74 | 0.71 | 2.06 |
| Range | | 1 – 11 | 1 – 11 | 1 – 6 | 1 – 3 | 1 – 4 | 1 – 11 |

*s* = standard deviation
*BC = birth control
†in years

the TOWs. The oral contraceptive pill ($N = 54; 67\%$) and the condom ($N = 26; 32\%$) were the most commonly mentioned methods. Only small percentages of teens (less than 5%), mentioned any of the other contraceptive methods available in the United States or Latin America (diaphragm, IUD, spermicides, Depo-Provera, rhythm, withdrawal, sterilization).

### Contraceptive Plans

Since the Teen Project focused on promoting contraceptive use to prevent a rapid repeat pregnancy, much of the work the TOWs did was to provide information and education about methods, to allay fears about side effects, to correct misconceptions about the safety of contraceptive methods, and to provide support and encouragement for consistent contraceptive use. As indicated above, the TOWs discovered that upon entry into this program the young mothers were relatively unfamiliar with contraceptive methods, and very few had used a method in the past. As part of the intervention protocol the TOWs provided information and demonstrations of contraceptive methods at the initial interview on the postpartum ward. The use of foam and condoms was demonstrated, and each teen left the hospital with a supply of foam and condoms for use in the interval between delivery and the postpartum appointment four to six weeks later. Sexual intercourse is generally discouraged by biomedical providers for four to six weeks after delivery. Among Latina women the *quarentena* (the traditional forty-day recovery period after childbirth that includes special food, rest, and sexual abstinence) is observed by many women (see Kay 1978). A significant proportion of the teens in this sample (31%), however, did have intercourse before they returned for their postpartum appointment. Although the risk of pregnancy is very low during this period, the risk of infection is generally thought to be higher than usual because the cervix can still be dilated. Thus, foam and condoms should prevent both infection and pregnancy if they are used.

After the education session on the postpartum ward, the young woman was asked whether she intended to contracept and what method she was considering. The majority of these young mothers indicated that they wanted to use a method of contraception postpartum (79%). Fourteen percent had no partner at the time and, therefore, were not in need of contraception; 6% were not sure; and only 1% said they did not plan to use a method (see Table 7.2). Of those who intended to use a method, over half (60%) said they wanted to use oral contraceptive pills, about one-quarter (27%) were not sure what method they wanted, 5% wanted foam and condoms,[2] 3% wanted another method, and 5% indicated they needed to discuss the matter with their partner before deciding. Most (74%) planned to begin using contraception after the postpartum appointment about four weeks after the baby's birth, but 18% said they would begin when they became sexually active again. There were virtually no differences among the language or cultural groups regarding contraceptive plans postpartum.

### Reproductive Plans

Almost half (46%) of the young mothers told the TOWs that they did not want to have any more children, 35% were unsure, and 19% indicated they did want more. Spanish speakers were more likely than English speakers to indicate they definitely did not want any more children (53% vs. 35%). Among those who did want to have more children (or who were unsure; $N = 88$), the mean number of additional children desired was 1.5 ($s = 1.2$, range 1–10).

The majority (65%) of those who wanted to have another child wanted to wait five or more years before having another (mean 4.4, $s = 1.4$ years). Only 10% wanted to have another child within two years of this birth. Thus, the goal of preventing a pregnancy for two years was consistent with the stated desires of most of the young mothers interviewed.

The average number of children desired[3] by these mothers was 1.9 ($s = 1.2$, range 1–11; see Table 7.2). The range was greater for English speakers than for Spanish speakers, but there was no difference in the mean desired family size. Among the cultural groups, the Central American–born teens had the highest mean number of desired children (2.3) and the widest range (1–11); Mexican-born teens had the lowest desired number (1.7) and an intermediate range (1–4); and U.S.-born teens had an intermediate desired number of children (2.0), but the smallest range (1–3). None of these differences were statistically significant, however.

### Return for the Postpartum Appointment

Of the 173 mothers interviewed on the postpartum ward, 143 (83%) returned to the clinic for their postpartum medical visit four weeks after the birth of their baby (see Table 7.3). Thus, at this point, 17% of the cases were lost to follow-up. While this is a high rate of loss to follow-up, comparison to the control group, among whom over one-third (36%) did not return for their appointments, suggests that the program was effective in attracting teen mothers into care at this first family planning visit. The difference in return rate between cases and controls was statistically significant (chi-square $= 10.5579$, $df = 1$, $p < .001$). The TOWs telephoned the project cases to remind them of their appointments. Controls were not called. This simple intervention reduced loss to follow-up at postpartum by about half. There

Table 7.3.    Mothers Returning for Postpartum Appointment

|  | Total | | English Speakers | Spanish Speakers | U.S. | Mexico | Central America |
|  | N | % | % | % | % | % | % |
|---|---|---|---|---|---|---|---|
| Case | 173 | 83 | 89 | 79 | 88 | 81 | 86 |
| Control | 99 | 64 | | | | | |

*Difference between case and control significant at p < .001

were no significant differences between English and Spanish speakers nor among the cultural groups regarding return for postpartum care.

### Living Arrangements Postpartum

Of the teen mothers who were cases and who came for their appointment, 84% were living at the same address given during the first interview about one month earlier, and 66% were still with the baby's father. Over half (55%) were receiving economic support from the baby's father; 29% from their own parents; 10% were supporting themselves; and a small proportion (6%) were receiving AFDC. Sixteen teens (12%) were attending school at the time of the appointment, and 64% of those not attending said they would like to return to school. Six teens (5%) were working. Most (83%) were staying home and caring for the new baby.

### Sexual Behavior Postpartum

At the postpartum visit the young women were asked their age at first menstruation and at first intercourse. The mean age at first menstruation for the teens was 12.2 ($s = 1.3$, range 9–15; $N = 138$) years and did not differ among the language or cultural groups. The mean age at first intercourse was 14.8 ($s = 1.2$, range 11–17; $N = 131$) years and, like age at first menstruation, did not differ among the groups. On the average, then, the young women in this sample had their first sexual intercourse about two and one-half years (mean 2.6, $s = 1.4$, range 0–6) after their first menstruation. Among the primiparous teens, the mean difference between age at first intercourse and age at first birth was about 1.2 years ($s = 0.2$, range 0–4), suggesting that pregnancy rapidly followed commencement of sexual activity and corroborating the low use of contraception prior to pregnancy among these young women.

Almost one-third ($N = 44$; 31%) of these young women had resumed having sexual intercourse by the time they came for their postpartum check-up. Of these, 68% had used a method of contraception, primarily foam and condoms (87%) or withdrawal (13%). Although the risk of pregnancy is quite low in the first weeks following birth, at the postpartum visit ten pregnancy tests were performed, two of which were positive. Six teens were diagnosed with a sexually transmitted infection (STI), primarily herpes, condyloma, and/or chlamydia, the most common STIs treated in the clinic. During the study period there was an epidemic of condyloma in L.A.

## Contraception Postpartum

Almost all of the teens (90%) wanted a method of contraception, and the remaining 10% intended to remain abstinent. Of those who wanted a contraceptive method, most (79%) wanted the oral contraceptive pill, 12% wanted to use foam and condoms, and 7% wanted some other method. Of those requesting oral contraceptives pills, 94% received them. Methods dispensed at the postpartum visit ($N = 109$) were: 81% oral contraceptive pills, 14% foam and condoms, and 4% some other method. One teen chose to remain abstinent.

Forty-one percent of the teens ($N = 58$) indicated they had special concerns or problems at this clinic visit. The most common psychosocial problems of these fifty-eight young mothers about one month after the birth were economic (35%), partner related (29%), related to a severely ill infant (9%), and family related (9%). Two teens (3%) indicated they were being physically abused, and four (7%) were being sexually abused. Three (5%) were gang-involved, and one had a partner who was in jail.

After the postpartum appointment, follow-up visits were made according to the medical protocol for the particular contraceptive method the teen chose and for any medical problems she might have had over the time she remained in the program. Overall, after the initial postpartum clinic visit, there were 332 clinic visits made by 105 of the teens. Of the original 173 teens interviewed, only 61% used the clinic after the postpartum clinic visit. Of these, the majority were for oral contraceptive pill refills and monitoring (45%) and other medical problems (29%). An additional 12% were for annual exams, 8% for pregnancy tests, 4% for method problems, and 2% for test of cure for STI treatment.

To evaluate the success of the program, the longitudinal charts and medical records of the teen mothers and the medical records of the controls were reviewed after one year to determine whether cases had avoided a repeat pregnancy better than controls. At this one-year follow-up we discovered an extremely high rate (87%) of loss to follow-up among the controls. Attempts to reach controls by phone and mail were unsuccessful, and the case-control design was abandoned.

### Program Retention

#### Loss to Follow-up at One Year

The majority of both cases (58%) and controls (87%) were lost to follow-up before one year of program participation (see Table 7.4). Significantly fewer cases than controls were lost to follow-up (chi-square = 23.614, $df$ = 1, $p$ < .0001), however, and on the average, the cases remained in the program about one and one-half months longer than the controls (mean 4.4 months vs. 1.9 months, $t$ = 4.2674, $df$ = 161.3, $p$ < .0001). Because of their longer retention in the program, the cases also had more clinic visits than the controls. The mean number of visits for the case group was 2.5 ($s$ = 2.0) and 1.2 ($s$ = 1.2) for the controls ($t$ = 6.5885, $df$ = 257.9, $p$ < .001).

Among the cases, there were no statistically significant language- or cultural-group differences regarding retention in the program even though a greater proportion of English speakers (63%) than Spanish speakers (54%) was lost to follow-up. Among the cultural groups, the Mexican-born teens had a greater proportion remaining in the program at the end of one year (47%) than either U.S.-born (35%) or Central American–born (33%) teens. Although these differences in retention are not statistically significant, they are suggestive of a better retention for Mexican-born teens.

There were no significant differences in length of time in the program between Mexican- and U.S.-born teens or between the U.S.- and Central American–born teens, but the Mexican-born teens remained in the program longer than the Central Americans. Although the overall model was significant, very little of the variance (8%) is explained by cultural-group affiliation ($F$ = 4.04, $p$ < .02, R-Square = .084).[4]

Among the cases not lost to follow-up, the mean number of clinic visits was 3.7 with a range of 1 to 9. This number includes the postpartum appointment and any other follow-up care the teen received in the clinic either for contraception or other medical care (for vaginal infection, STI, etc.) and roughly translated to one visit every three months.

#### Loss to Follow-up at Two Years

Loss to follow-up in the two-year follow-up group is presented in Table 7.5, although the number of teens eligible for follow-up after two years is quite small. Seventy-eight of the cases and 60 controls who entered the program

Table 7.4.    Retention in Teen Program

| Variable | Total | | English Speakers | Spanish Speakers | U.S. | Mexico | Central America |
|---|---|---|---|---|---|---|---|
| | N | % | % | % | % | % | % |
| | | | Lost by One Year Follow-up* | | | | |
| Case | 172 | 58 | 63 | 54 | 65 | 53 | 67 |
| Control | 99 | 87 | | | | | |
| | | | Mean Number of Months in Program at Loss* | | | | |
| Case | 92 | 4.4 | 4.0 | 4.8 | 3.5 | 5.5 | 2.7** |
| s | | 4.5 | 4.3 | 5.6 | 3.2 | 5.0 | 1.9 |
| Range | | 0–14 | 0–12 | 0–14 | 0–8 | 0–14 | 0–9 |
| Control | 75 | 1.9 | | | | | |
| s | | 3.1 | | | | | |
| Range | | 0–12 | | | | | |
| | | | Mean Number of Clinic Visits* | | | | |
| Case | 172 | 2.5 | 2.3 | 2.6 | 2.1 | 2.8 | 1.9 |
| s | | 2.0 | 2.1 | 1.9 | 1.8 | 2.1 | 1.6 |
| Range | | 0–9 | 0–9 | 0–7 | 0–5 | 0–9 | 0–7 |
| Control | 94 | 1.2 | | | | | |
| s | | 1.3 | | | | | |
| Range | | 0–6 | | | | | |

$s$ = standard deviation
* Case/control difference significant at $p < .001$
** Mexican/Central American difference significant at $p < .05$

Table 7.5.    Loss to Follow-up in the Two Year Sample

| Variable | Total | | English Speakers | Spanish Speakers | U.S. | Mexico | Central America |
|---|---|---|---|---|---|---|---|
| | N | % | % | % | % | % | % |
| Lost to Follow-up (Two Year Sample, $N = 26$) | | | | | | | |
| Case | 24 | 33 | 40 | 32 | 33 | 33 | 0 |
| Control | 2 | 50 | | | | | |
| Mean Number of Months in Program at Loss | | | | | | | |
| Case | 6 | 16.5 | 15.5 | 17.0 | 15.5 | 17.0 | 0 |
| s | | 2.6 | 3.5 | 2.5 | 3.5 | 2.5 | — |
| Range | | 13–19 | 13–18 | 14–19 | 13–18 | 14–19 | — |
| Control | 1 | 16.0 | | | | | |

$s$ = standard deviation

between April and December 1989 were eligible for the two-year follow-up in December 1991 when the evaluation was performed. Of these, only 24 cases (31%) and two controls (3%) were still active at the beginning of the second-year follow-up period. Of those who were active, half of the controls and one-third of the cases were lost to follow-up during the second year. Only 21% of the two-year sample cases remained in the program for two years, and virtually all of the controls were lost to follow-up.

These results suggest that variables other than cultural group and acculturation are important for retention in care. Whenever possible, the TOWs asked the teen during telephone follow-up why she discontinued care. Among the cases for whom information about the reason for loss to follow-up was available ($N = 81$; 82% of those lost), 10% had moved (half back to their country of origin), 11% had moved out of the clinic's catchment area, and 12% had a repeat pregnancy they were continuing to term and were not in need of family planning care.

Thus, legitimate reasons for loss to follow-up, such as moving (21%) and repeat pregnancy (12%), accounted for about one-third of the loss to follow-up. Some, however, chose to discontinue care (20%) for their own reasons, which they did not share with the TOWs. The majority of those lost to follow-up (47%), however, simply could not be contacted by the TOWs. Telephone numbers were either incorrect or disconnected, and follow-up letters sent to the address given by the teen were returned to the clinic as undeliverable.

The very high proportion of loss to follow-up could be interpreted as evidence that the program was not worth the effort in terms of cost-benefit, because it was quite expensive, over $100,000 per year for TOWs alone, not including the cost of medical care or office space. Moreover, the high loss to follow-up in the control group effectively precluded case-control comparison of the primary outcome measure, repeat pregnancy, thus eliminating any hope of proving program efficacy in its primary goal. Yet, the greater retention of cases suggests that the program had a positive, if limited, short-term effect in retaining teen mothers in family planning care. This is the first step toward pregnancy prevention.

Although we had anticipated loss to follow-up in the project design, our estimates of 25% to 30%[5] were much lower than those actually found with this population. Recent research on contraceptive discontinuation in a multiethnic adolescent family planning population indicates that 58% of Latina teens did not return for their three-to-four-month oral contraceptive pill follow-up appointments compared to 44% of white and 45% of African American teens (Wiemann and Berenson 1993). Our results are very similar to this—58% lost to follow-up at one year, with a mean of 4.4 months in the program at loss to follow-up. Over the course of the project, it became increasingly clear that follow-up by telephone and mail assumed a stability in residence and phone service that is common in middle-class populations but only achieved by a small proportion of the teens in this sample.

Intermittent telephone service was a significant problem, and telephones were frequently disconnected for varying periods of time.[6] It was not unusual, for example, for a phone to be disconnected for several weeks or months and then to be reconnected. As Blanca notes, "They don't have enough to pay the bill, so it's disconnected. Then, when they get a little ahead, maybe it's four months later, they connect it again."

Many teens were lost during these "down times" in their telephone service only to be "found" again later when service was restored. Many of the teens also used friends' or relatives' telephones as message phones because they did not have a telephone where they lived. Although letters were used as a back-up for those with no telephone, this was less than adequate since many teens did not know their address or gave an incomplete or false one.

Another factor in loss to follow-up was the mobility of the population. Many of these young women moved from household to household. Blanca referred to them as "gypsies" and described a typical scenario:

> First she lives with her mother, then there are too many people in that house so she goes to an aunt for a while, then the aunt gets tired of the baby crying and she goes to live with the baby's father's family, then they have a fight and she goes back to her mother, but her mother makes her baby-sit her brothers and sisters and she feels too tied down there so goes to live with her *cuñada* [baby's father's sister], and then she gets back with the father, or she goes off to Mexico for three months or forever, or the grandmother's sick, or up north with her boyfriend to pick fruit. Sometimes they go to other states and come back six months later, pregnant. Sometimes they just go back to Mexico and don't come back. Often we just don't know. No one knows where she went, she's just gone.

An additional barrier is the fear of deportation among undocumented teens or those who reside with other undocumented persons. Many undocumented women are afraid to use health or social services to which their baby is entitled as a United States citizen for fear of being found by the Immigration and Naturalization Service and sent back to their country of citizenship. This results in provision of incorrect telephone and address information to health providers and also to use of health services only in emergency situations. As Carmen notes:

> Sometimes you won't see them for months. One of my girls, I couldn't get a hold of her for her pill check . . . telephone disconnected, letters all

came back, and I black-dotted her [closed the case], and she came back in because she had condyloma so bad she couldn't walk.

The TOWs feel that the undocumented, recently arrived teens are the most likely to "disappear." Since legal residence is not required for medical care, and the TOWs know the question is sensitive, they pointedly do not ask about legal residence, and no quantification of this hypothesis is possible for this sample.

The other group of teens likely to be lost to follow-up are those who are involved in drugs or gangs. As Alicia notes, "They'll [drug users] just lie to you . . . tell you anything to keep you from knowing where they're at. They know how to use the system and know how to stay out of it, too."

The lack of association of language and ethnicity with retention in the program seems inconsistent with the TOWs' comments offered above. Interviews with the TOWs suggest that the U.S.-born teens were more likely to be from dysfunctional families involved in generational poverty, drugs, and gangs. The Spanish speakers, on the other hand, roughly fell into two categories: those who were recently arrived and undocumented or those who had lived here longer and were a more stable group both geographically and socially. This latter group represents less recent immigrants who had probably been to school in the United States; who were from families often referred to as the working poor; and who had not yet been able to accumulate the resources to move out of inner-city East Los Angeles to more suburban Latino communities. It is possible that the higher proportion of Mexican-born teens retained in the program may reflect this more stable immigrant population, although it is not possible to be certain from these data.

Poverty was also implicated as a major factor in loss to follow-up because it leads to other difficulties of daily living, including transportation problems, time-allocation difficulties, a low priority attached to clinic attendance relative to other more pressing needs, and the rather high residential mobility for these young women and their babies. As Blanca tells it:

> [They] work long hours at low-paying jobs with no benefits and can barely manage the costs of the new baby. Sometimes it's the choice between a gallon of milk and the bus fare to go to the clinic . . . then if you take the bus you have to drag the baby with you and if there are other children, too . . . it's just too much. I forgot what that was [like].

Thus, one of the interventions on which the project was based, intensive follow-up, could not be achieved to the degree desired, and follow-up frequently became dependent on the teens' keeping in touch with the TOWs, just as it is in regular family planning care. This aspect of project design did not "fit" the population served. It was based on a model that presumed ease in maintaining contact with young mothers via telephone or mail. Once this became apparent, we investigated the possibility of the TOWs making home visits to the young mothers, but this was not an option because of legal restrictions on hospital employees. Issues of personal safety were also of concern. However, given both the transiency of the population and the vested interests by some that their whereabouts not be known, it is not at all clear that the ability to make home visits would have proved useful. In sum, the project was not able to overcome the difficulties in maintaining contact with the young mothers—contact on which the intervention depended.

## Repeat Pregnancy

Information about repeat pregnancy within the one- and two-year follow-up periods is given in Table 7.6. It is important to remember that information on this variable is missing for over half of the sample after one year and for over three-quarters after two years due to loss to follow-up. Although data for the control group are presented, high loss to follow-up effectively precludes valid comparison of cases to controls on the pregnancy outcome variables.

Among the cases, seventeen teens had one repeat pregnancy and two had two repeat pregnancies, for a total of twenty-one repeat pregnancies among nineteen teens during the one-year follow-up period. In the two-year follow-up period, only five cases had a repeat pregnancy (only one control was left at the time). Four teens had a pregnancy in the first six months of the second year and one in the final six months. Of the teens remaining in the program for two years, only three had had a repeat pregnancy during both the one- and two-year follow-up periods.

In all, then, 22% of the teens had a repeat pregnancy during the one- and two-year follow-up periods. The repeat-pregnancy rate (i.e., number of pregnancies divided by number of teens) was 24% in the first follow-up period and 22% in the second.[7] Our one-year rate is greater than the 17% probability of repeat pregnancy within one year for all teenage mothers in the United States and similar to the 21% estimate for teen mothers below 150% of poverty (Ford 1983). Mott (1986), however, documented that rapid repeat birth is more common among Latina than among African American or white teen mothers. For Latinas who had a first birth when they were 16 or younger, the repeat-birth rate within twenty-four months of the first birth was 39% (vs. 30% for African Americans and 21% for whites); for those having a first birth at age 17, the repeat rate was 27% (vs. 20% for African Americans and 23% for whites). This pattern was also apparent among all Latina age groups (i.e., ages 19–22 at first birth) in the sample (Mott 1986).

Table 7.6.    Repeat Pregnancy within One and Two Years

| Variable | Total N | Total % | English Speakers N | English Speakers % | Spanish Speakers N | Spanish Speakers % | U.S. N | U.S. % | Mexico N | Mexico % | Central America N | Central America % |
|---|---|---|---|---|---|---|---|---|---|---|---|---|
| **Repeat Pregnancy within Six Months** | | | | | | | | | | | | |
| Case (88)* | 15 | 17 | 3 | 11 | 12 | 20 | 1 | 13 | 10 | 16 | 3 | 18 |
| Control (11) | 1 | 9 | | | | | | | | | | |
| **Any Repeat Pregnancy within One Year** | | | | | | | | | | | | |
| Case (87) | 19 | 22 | 7 | 26 | 12 | 20 | 4 | 50 | 11 | 18 | 4 | 24 |
| Control (11) | 2 | 18 | | | | | | | | | | |
| **Repeat Pregnancy during Second Year** | | | | | | | | | | | | |
| Case (23) | 5 | 22 | 2 | 40 | 3 | 17 | 2 | 33 | 3 | 18 | 0 | — |
| Control (1) | 0 | 0 | | | | | | | | | | |

* Numbers in parentheses denote total number in group
N = number of teens with a repeat pregnancy
Percentage is percentage of total in group

Thus, the repeat-pregnancy rate among those remaining in the Teen Program was lower than the repeat-birth rate among Latinas in Mott's study.

Of the teens in the one-year sample with repeat pregnancies, eight had decided to continue the pregnancy, five to terminate, and six were undecided at the follow-up. Of those who became pregnant during the second year, three were planning to terminate, and information for the remaining two was unknown. Based on the teen mothers' intention about pregnancy resolution at follow-up, we estimate that about one-third of teens with repeat pregnancies decided to continue their pregnancies, one-third to terminate, and one-third were undecided or the information was not available at follow-up. Thus, the repeat-birth rate is likely to be lower than the repeat-pregnancy rate.

Our repeat-pregnancy rate was similar to national rates of repeat pregnancy for all teens. Compared to the repeat-birth rates for Latina teens aged 17 and under two years after a first birth, however, teens remaining in our program were likely to have lower rates of repeat birth. However, the high attrition among cases dilutes the strength of these findings, since teens who remained in the Teen Project were probably more highly motivated to prevent pregnancy.

The lack of greater impact was particularly upsetting to the TOWs. They were really striving to "make a difference" in these young women's lives. Two of the TOWs had been teenage mothers themselves, and all four had come back to East L.A. to give something back to their community. They wanted to help the young mothers prevent a rapid repeat pregnancy, return to school, and become economically self-sufficient.

Was the project a failure? From a research standpoint, the project, as designed, was a disaster. High attrition rates precluded the case-control design and biased repeat-pregnancy rates in our favor (i.e., teens remaining in the project were probably more motivated to prevent pregnancy). Yet our cases did no better than teens nationwide and had one-year repeat-pregnancy rates similar to teens below 150% of poverty.

Mott's (1986) data provided a more relevant comparison group, since, according to him, "[They were likely to] represent a relatively unacculturated subgroup, with more traditional attitudes toward motherhood and higher education for women" (p. 11). Mott, however, was measuring repeat birth at twenty-four months, and we were measuring repeat pregnancy, making comparison imprecise. Given that gestation lasts about nine months, most of the teens in his sample would have had to become pregnant within fifteen months of the first birth. Compared to his repeat-birth rates of 39% for Latinas aged 16 or under and 27% for those aged 17, our rates of repeat pregnancy at one (24%) and two (22%) years were lower. Considering that some of the teens with repeat pregnancies were planning to terminate their pregnancies, our repeat-birth rate would probably be much lower. We can never know whether this was due to program effects or bias in the sample due to attrition.

The Teen Project was able to increase return for postpartum care and to retain case teens in care longer, as compared to the controls. This is especially important in the context of the transiency of the population. Maintaining contact with poor teen mothers, many of whom were in the United States illegally, is difficult in the best of circumstances, but even more so in urban Los Angeles. That so many of the cases remained in the program despite transportation and other difficulties is truly a tribute to the TOWs and their hard work and dedication and to the young women themselves.

From a service standpoint, the project was very successful. Many individual teens were helped by the TOWs. Some left abusive relationships, others were helped to find housing, still others were referred to emergency food resources. Some teens had their first job in our clinic. One teen mother even brought her sister in for birth control before she became sexually active. These were small successes, but they are not trivial for the lives of individual young women.

Was the project a success? It depends how success is defined and measured.

## CHAPTER EIGHT

# Contraceptive Use
## The Intervening Variable

In general, compared to white and African American teens, Latina teens know less about birth control and are less likely to use birth control at first intercourse, have lower rates of contraceptive use overall, and initiate contraceptive use a longer time after becoming sexually active. They tend to have conservative attitudes and behaviors regarding sexuality and gender roles. If they become pregnant, they are less likely to abort than to carry to term. After the first birth, however, contraceptive use becomes more acceptable for child spacing. These generalizations from the literature (see Chapter 2) hold for the teen mothers interviewed on the postpartum ward. About half knew about birth control, but only 13% had ever used it in the past. None had opted to terminate the pregnancy even though 63% were unintended. Most (79%) wanted to use a contraceptive method postpartum (another 14% were abstinent) and to wait several years before having another child.

The Teen Project was developed to intervene during the postpartum period to encourage and facilitate contraceptive use and thereby help the young mothers delay subsequent pregnancy. It should have been easy. Contraception was now more culturally appropriate, and sex was no longer taboo. The majority of the young women were married or living with their partners, and as mothers and wives, were now expected to have sexual relationships with their partners. The Project should have been able to reduce repeat pregnancy to almost nothing. Why did so many of the young mothers have a repeat pregnancy? In order to answer this question, we have to look at contraceptive use, the intervening variable between the project intervention and the outcome measure (pregnancy).

### Contraceptive Use over Time

In the evaluation design, we chose an easily measured event (repeat pregnancy documented in the medical record) as our outcome variable, assuming that it would be any contraceptive use facilitated by the TOWs that reduced the repeat-pregnancy rate among cases as compared to controls. However, the data on contraceptive use were based on the method documented in the medical record and may have had little to do with actual use of that method or the quality and consistency of use.[1]

## Problems Measuring Contraceptive Use

Tracking of actual contraceptive use in this group over time was quite difficult because of problems tapping the relevant information from the medical record and the longitudinal project record. At each clinic visit, the TOWs would note the contraceptive method the teen said she was using or had received at that visit, yet in the time intervening between contacts there were many possibilities regarding actual use. For example, the teen could use the method correctly and continuously, sometimes use the method, take the method but never use it, stop using the method because of side effects, give it to a friend to use, and so on. The range of possibilities is large and varied and was rarely documented in the medical record. Even the longitudinal records, much better sources of more individualized behavior, were incomplete in this regard. It was only through interviews with TOWs (and sometimes reading medical record notes) that one could get a sense of the vast difference between receiving a method at a clinic visit and actually using it.

## Method Change

Table 8.1 provides a summary of methods the teen mothers received from the clinic at the postpartum appointment, and at the visits closest to six, twelve, and twenty-four months after the entry birth. Oral contraceptive pills were clearly the most widely utilized method at all four time periods. Overall, 74% of the young mothers received oral contraceptive pills at the postpartum visit, 67% continued with them at six months, 63% at twelve months, and 68% at twenty-four months. The proportion using oral contraceptive pills declined slightly over the follow-up period with a concomitant rise in intrauterine device use and abstinence. Foam and condoms were the second most widely used method at all time periods. At the six- and twelve-month follow-ups, there was a small shift to use of no medical method, although traditional methods not documented in the chart (e.g., withdrawal and rhythm) could have been used.

Although the overall group shift toward less effective methods over time is a valuable indicator of changes in patterns of contraceptive use that might affect repeat pregnancy, the history of individual method switching over time is of more interest for two reasons. First, in the short run, high rates of method switching may be associated with higher risk of repeat pregnancy.

Table 8.1.    Contraceptive Methods Used over Time *

| Method | Postpartum | | 6 Months | | 12 Months | | 24 Months | |
|---|---|---|---|---|---|---|---|---|
| | N | % | N | % | N | % | N | % |
| Total | 140 | | 131 | | 97 | | 25 | |
| Oral contraceptive pill | 103 | 74 | 88 | 67 | 61 | 63 | 17 | 68 |
| Foam and condoms | 31 | 22 | 25 | 19 | 14 | 14 | 6 | 24 |
| Intrauterine device | 1 | 1 | 4 | 3 | 3 | 3 | 2 | 8 |
| Diaphragm | 2 | 1 | 2 | 2 | 1 | 1 | 0 | — |
| Abstinence | 2 | 1 | 7 | 5 | 5 | 5 | 0 | — |
| Other | 1 | 1 | 0 | — | 0 | — | 0 | — |
| None | 0 | — | 5 | 4 | 13 | 13 | 0 | — |

* Percentages do not always sum to 100 due to rounding

Second, in the long run, shifts toward use of more effective methods over time, a common pattern among adolescents (Zelnik et al. 1981), might lower the rates of repeat pregnancy. Both factors appear to be operating in this sample. Among 106 teens who came to their postpartum appointment and had at least one other clinic visit, a large proportion (41%) switched contraceptive methods one or more times during the time they were in the project. Teens with higher method-switching rates (i.e., those who changed methods two or more times) were about five times more likely to have a repeat pregnancy than those with low switching rates (those who did not change at all or changed only once). Among the high switch-rate group, 46% had a repeat pregnancy compared to only 8% among the low switch rate group (chi-square = 8.03, $df = 1$, $p < .01$). Thus, in the short run, method switching appears to be detrimental to prevention of repeat pregnancy in this group.

Over the long haul, however, there was a tendency for the teens remaining in the project longer (five or more visits) to shift to use of highly effective medical methods of contraception (oral contraceptive pills and intrauterine devices).[2] For example, 85% to 100% of the teens with more than five clinic visits were using oral contraceptive pills compared to about 70% initially. This change probably reflects both the greater commitment of teens remaining in family planning care to avoiding a subsequent pregnancy and their greater familiarity with contraception.

It is interesting to note that the proportion using foam and condoms, abstinence, or no method (21–31%) is roughly similar to the proportion who had a repeat pregnancy (22%). In fact, a significantly greater proportion of teens who were using a less effective method (foam and condoms, diaphragm, abstinence, or nothing) at the clinic visit closest to the twelve-month visit (when most of the repeat pregnancies occurred) had a repeat

Table 8.2.    Percentage with Repeat Pregnancy by Contraceptive Method Reported at 12-Month Follow-up

| | | | Not | | Lowest* | |
| | Pregnant | | Pregnant | | Expected | Typical |
| Method | N | % | N | % | N | % |
| --- | --- | --- | --- | --- | --- | --- |
| Oral contraceptive pill | 6 | 10 | 57 | 90 | 0.1–0.5 | 3 |
| Intrauterine device | 0 | — | 3 | 100 | 0.8–2 | 2 |
| Condom and foam | 2 | 20 | 8 | 80 | 2.0† | 12† |
| | | | | | 3.0† | 21† |
| Diaphragm | 0 | — | 1 | 100 | 6.0 | 18 |
| Abstinence | 0 | — | 4 | 100 | | |
| Nothing | 10 | 77 | 3 | 23 | 85.0 | 85 |
| Medical | 6 | 9 | 60 | 91 | | |
| Nonmedical | 13 | 45 | 16 | 55 | | |

*Percentage of women experiencing pregnancy in one year, lowest expected and typical failure rates (Hatcher et al., 1990, pp. 134–135)
† Rates are for condom without spermicide and spermicide without condom

pregnancy than those using a more effective method (oral contraceptive pills, intrauterine device). The proportion of teens experiencing a pregnancy with each method at twelve months is provided in Table 8.2 and roughly approximates the typical failure rate of the different methods, except for oral contraceptive pill use, which was higher.

This is not particularly surprising because typical failure rates are calculated based on pregnancy rates among typical users during one year of use. Although the lowest expected failure rate for foam and condoms is quite low (2–3%) and is similar to that of the intrauterine device and oral contraceptive pills, the typical failure rates of both foam and condoms are quite a bit higher than those of either the intrauterine device or oral contraceptive pills. Thus, in this population group, repeat-pregnancy prevention may be dependent more on fostering the early and continued use of highly effective contraceptive methods, such as oral contraceptive pills and intrauterine devices, than on fostering contraceptive use in general. Case data suggest that the high rate of repeat pregnancy among oral contraceptive pill acceptors was primarily due to method discontinuance rather than method failure.

Several problematic issues arise from the data presented above. First, some teen mothers may be less motivated than others to prevent a subsequent pregnancy, and hence, be less motivated to use contraception. Second, even among those who are motivated, use of the most effective medical contraceptive methods may be problematic either because they are medically contraindicated or because of individual or cultural preferences discouraging use of medical methods, especially oral contraceptive pills. Third, none of the methods is 100% effective in preventing pregnancy, and efficacy is often dependent on consistency of use and diligence on the part of the young mother. This is especially true for oral contraceptive pills and foam and condoms, the two most widely accepted methods in this group. Thus, many factors associated with contraceptive prescription and use affect pregnancy prevention.

The quantitative data suggest that teens who use highly effective methods of contraception, who do not change methods more than once, and who actually use their method (inferred not documented) tend to be more successful in preventing rapid repeat pregnancy than those teens who use less effective methods, change methods often, or use their method incorrectly (inferred from failure rates).

### Factors Affecting Contraceptive Use [3]

Because these data tell us little about the reasons for the behaviors documented, the TOWs and I began a more qualitative investigation to find out what factors affected individual teens' use of contraception. It is important to keep in mind that most of the teens in this sample chose oral contraceptive pills, and thus, much of the information that follows is applicable particularly to this method.

The TOWs thought that the young mothers refused or discontinued contraceptive use primarily for four reasons: (1) side effects and fear of the consequences of medical methods; (2) the regimen and protocol for oral contraceptive pill use, which necessitates frequent clinic returns for medical supervision (at three months, six months, and one year for first-time users); (3) any disruption of the sexual relationship with the baby's father whether it is likely to be permanent or temporary; and (4) her mother or partner prohibiting contraceptive use. The first two factors apply particularly to medical methods. The second set apply to any method.

### Medical Methods:
### Side Effects and Medical Protocol

With respect to fears about health consequences, Blanca notes:

> They're afraid to take the pill because some aunt got cancer and her mother told her it was from *la píldora* (the pill). . . . Usually we can convince them it's safe—especially when I say I was on it for five years.

Experience of any untoward symptoms, regardless of whether they are side effects from the method, is a real concern for these young women, as Carmen tells us:

I'd say half of my kids who stop it [the pill] do it in the first month they take it 'cause they get headaches or something and they're afraid of getting something worse. . . . Calling them up about two weeks into it helps to reassure them it's OK. Those symptoms are only temporary and will go away when their body adjusts to it.

Thus, the TOWs believe that education can play an important role in facilitating the use of medical methods of contraception for these young women, but it must be provided on a continuing basis to counteract the negative image the pill has in the Latino community.

Carolina's case illustrates how side effects led her to discontinue oral contraceptive pill use.

### Carolina, side effects

Carolina had just turned 16 and had delivered her second child when she was interviewed on the postpartum ward. She was from Nicaragua and had been in the United States for six years. She spoke some English but preferred Spanish. Carolina was in seventh grade when she dropped out of school because of her first pregnancy. Her first child was born in June when she was 13 years old. She took oral contraceptive pills at her postpartum visit but stopped using them because they "made her sick." Nine months later (in February) she terminated a subsequent pregnancy. Both pregnancies were from the same man, a 22-year-old whom Carolina regarded as her boyfriend. They had no plans to marry. Carolina lives with her family and they rely on AFDC for economic support. Carolina has never worked. She would like to go back to school but feels she can't with the responsibilities of caring for her two children.

Another important consideration regarding oral contraceptive pill use among these teens is that the regimen for use—taking pills every day at the same time of day—and the protocol for medical follow-up that requires numerous clinic visits (at three, six, and twelve months) do not fit nicely into the lifestyles of many of these young women, for whom motherhood, poverty, substance use, sexual abuse, physical abuse, and the uncertainties in daily living make consistency difficult to achieve.

Sylvia's case (first presented in Chapter 6) provides an example.

### Sylvia, lifestyle issues and residential transiency

Recall that Sylvia had planned her pregnancy and received early and continued prenatal care but delivered a low birth weight baby. Her lifestyle—multiple sexual partners, history of condyloma, and a partner involved in drugs and gangs—tagged her at high risk for STIs.

Sylvia's phone was often disconnected, and she moved several times.

She frequently failed her appointments and never used the pills she received. Her inability to comply with the oral contraceptive pill regimen placed her at risk for repeat pregnancy. Lack of a stable home, income, and someone to help her care for the baby seem to be the primary impediments to clinical follow-up for Sylvia.

Although Sylvia's case is extreme, even normal activities of daily living can make clinic return difficult, as Carmen tells us:

When they get back into school or get a job, they can't be taking off to come in and get their refills or [STI] check. Sometimes she'll call and say she ran out because she couldn't come in, and now she thinks she's pregnant.

Also of consideration are the transportation difficulties young teens may face in the Los Angeles metropolitan area, as Carmen notes:

Some of my teens, they baby-sit other kids to make money, and they can't take off work to come to the clinic. Or he can't take off work to drive her, and she doesn't know how to take the bus. It's a long way to come for a lot of them.

Amelia's case illustrates well many of the complexities of life and contraception.

### Amelia, young teen

Amelia was interviewed in December 1989 when she delivered her first child, a boy, at the age of 13. Amelia had come to the United States with her family from El Salvador three years before. She was in seventh grade when she got pregnant by her boyfriend, who was 20 years old. At the time, he was a security guard and had only completed seventh grade. She moved in with him during her pregnancy. Amelia knew about birth control but had never used it. She said she thought she couldn't get pregnant because she had been having sex for four months without becoming pregnant. Although neither she nor her boyfriend had planned to have a baby, she was happy when she found out she was pregnant. She had her first prenatal visit five months into the pregnancy and delivered a 2,400-gram infant three weeks before her estimated due date. The TOW's notes stated: "[Amelia] has a very good support system at home. She will be attending school. Patient is positive about using a BCM [birth control method]."

Amelia chose the minipill at her postpartum appointment because she was breast-feeding. In March she switched to combined oral contraceptive pills. In June she was complaining of nausea from the pill and missed an appointment because she had to work. She said that in order to cover the gap until she could come to the clinic she bought two cycles of pills from a woman she knew. In November 1990, Amelia was 15 years old and three months pregnant by a different man. In February 1991, she still had not gone for prenatal care and she was referred to a high-risk clinic and to a pregnant-teen program.

In March 1991 she was "found" on the postpartum ward. Amelia had had an emergency cesarean. Her second baby was born at twenty-four–twenty-six weeks, weighed 760 grams, and died the same day. A week later Amelia was diagnosed with herpes.

Amelia chose to use oral contraceptive pills at her postpartum appointment and has been a consistent user since April 1991. She is living with the first baby's father, and she is in school and plans to graduate and maybe go on to college.

It is also important to recognize that contraception may not be needed in every case, as Rosa's case (first presented in Chapter 6) suggests.

### Rosa, abstinent

Rosa's pregnancy was a result of rape, and although she received prenatal care, she delivered a very low birth weight infant with multiple medical problems. Although she chose oral contraceptive pills at her postpartum visit, she failed to comply with the follow-up regimen for two reasons: (1) she found clinic return difficult due to her baby's medical problems, and (2) she did not have a sexual partner and was abstinent.

Rosa's case illustrates a lack of fit between the project's objectives and the life of this young woman. Since follow-up was based on contraceptive protocols, abstinent teens tended to be peripheral to the main focus of the project and also tended to view their own involvement as a waste of time.

If oral contraceptive pills appear to be problematic, the question to ask is why they are prescribed so often. Medical providers at our clinic, and nationally, rely primarily on oral contraceptive pills for teenagers because of their high effectiveness. The teens in our project seemed to prefer oral contraceptive pills to the other methods available. The alternative methods were primarily barrier methods (spermicides, condoms, diaphragms, contraceptive sponge), which are coitus dependent. The literature on contraceptive acceptability suggests that Latinas, in general, prefer coitus-independent methods because of issues of female modesty about touching the genitals and the association of condom use with prostitutes (Marin et al. 1981).

Thus, the oral contraceptive pill becomes almost the only culturally and medically acceptable method available[4] for these young mothers. While the intrauterine device has potential for this population, it is medically contraindicated for teens because of the risk of infection and possible subsequent infertility. Only older, multiparous teens who have only one sexual partner are likely to receive an intrauterine device in American clinics. Although foam and condoms are the second most commonly received method of contraception in our group, it must be noted that they are routinely distributed as back-up measures when the teen chooses no other method of contraception or when medical considerations make it necessary to delay initiation of oral contraceptive pill use (e.g., waiting for the menses before beginning or resuming oral contraceptive pill use) or to discontinue oral contraceptive pill use for medical reasons (e.g., elevated blood pressure or other emergent problem). The actual extent of use of the foam and condoms dispensed is not known, although the repeat-pregnancy rate with the method is higher than the typical failure rate, suggesting that a significant proportion do not use the method.

### Attitudes toward Contraceptive Methods

An exploratory study comparing teens' and providers' attitudes toward the various contraceptive methods was carried out in the summer of 1992 using the same methods described in Chapter 5 for the study of women's roles and life events.[5] Twenty-eight teens and thirteen family planning care providers (three nurse practitioners, eight family planning counselors [including all the TOWs and the ward outreach worker], a nurse administrator, and a health educator) free-sorted sixteen contraceptive methods (see Table 8.3). The multidimensional scaling plots (see Figure 8.1) suggest that there was much greater conceptual agreement about the methods among the providers than among the teens.

The providers had three relatively tight clusters of methods: (1) the highly effective medical methods in the upper left-hand corner, (2) the barrier methods in the upper right-hand corner, and (3) natural, or traditional, methods requiring no "paraphernalia" at the bottom center of the plot. In fact, the providers labeled their piles in just this way. The medical methods were referred to variously as "more permanent, safe, little risk of pregnancy, more reliable, sure bets, most effective," and so on. One provider broke this cluster into subclusters based on how the methods worked (i.e., hormonal methods, intrauterine devices, and surgical methods), and several included ideas of permanency of effect, but the dominant underlying dimensions of classification were clearly related to effectiveness and to mode of use (natural, medical, barrier).

The two-dimensional multidimensional scaling plot for the teens was

Table 8.3.    English and Spanish Names of the Contraceptive Methods Used in
Pile Sorts and Ranking Exercises

| Code # | English | Spanish |
|---|---|---|
| 1 | Depo-Provera injections | Depo-Provera *inyecciones* |
| 2 | sponge | *esponja anticonceptiva* |
| 3 | spermicidal jelly/cream | *jalea/crema anticonceptiva* |
| 4 | diaphragm | *diafragma* |
| 5 | NORPLANT | NORPLANT/*aparato al brazo* |
| 6 | Intrauterine device (IUD) | *el aparato/anillo (DUI)* |
| 7 | oral contraceptives (the pill) | *pastillas anticonceptivas (la píldora)* |
| 8 | spermicidal foam | *espuma anticonceptiva* |
| 9 | condom | *condón* |
| 10 | rhythm/calendar | *ritmo/calendario* |
| 11 | natural family planning (temperature and mucous) | *planificación natural (temperatura y moco)* |
| 12 | withdrawal/pull out | *retiro/él me cuida* |
| 13 | abstinence (not having sex) | *abstinencia (no tener relaciones)* |
| 14 | sterilization | *la esterilización/operación* |
| 15 | nothing/no method | *nada/no usar nada/ningún método* |
| 16 | suppositories | *supositorios/óvulos* |

similar to that for the providers, and the correlation between the two was .74. The stress level of .16, however, suggested that a three-dimensional solution might better represent these data (Borgatti 1992). The three-dimensional multidimensional scaling plot for teens reduced the stress to an acceptable level (.10; see Figure 8.2), suggesting that the teens were using at least three underlying classification dimensions while sorting the birth control choices.

The three-dimensional plot suggests that the teens have six different clusters: (1) Depo-Provera, sterilization, abstinence, and NORPLANT (positive B quadrant); (2) natural family planning, rhythm, and withdrawal (negative B quadrant); (3) sponge, condoms, foam, and jelly (positive A, C, D quadrants) and diaphragm (negative A quadrant); (4) suppositories and intrauterine devices (negative A quadrant); (5) no method; and (6) oral contraceptive pills (almost on the plane in B and D quadrants, respectively, which might best be understood as standing alone).

The text data suggest that the teens were using four underlying classification dimensions, the same two used by the providers: efficacy and mode of use; and two additional dimensions: personal familiarity with method and whether the teen would actually use the method herself, dimensions that were not salient in the provider sorts.

The first dimension, that of efficacy, usually was apparent only at the

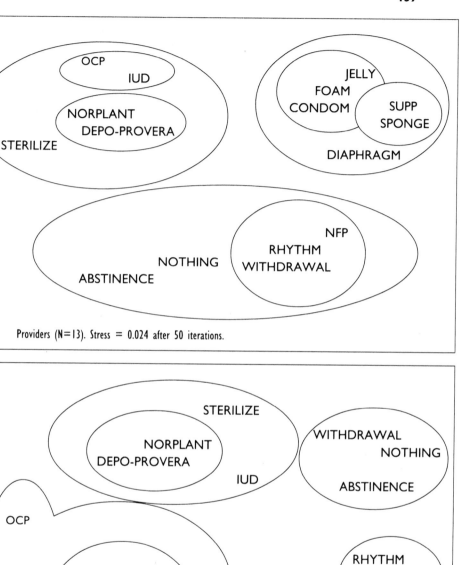

Providers (N=13). Stress = 0.024 after 50 iterations.

Teens (N=28). Stress = 0.162 after 22 iterations.

Figure 8.1.  Two-dimensional multidimensional scaling plots of providers' and teens' free sort of contra-ceptive methods

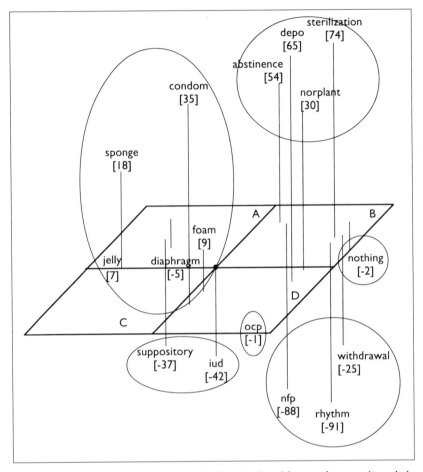

Figure 8.2.    Three-dimensional multidimensional scaling plot of teens' free sort of contraceptive methods N = 28. Stress 0.10 after 28 iterations.

most effective pole: "*son los mejores* (these are the best), best for not getting pregnant" and were used with the most effective medical methods
(oral contraceptive pills, NORPLANT, the intrauterine device, and sterilization). Occasionally there would be some labeling of methods at the
other extreme, but this was much less common and used primarily with
rhythm, withdrawal, and nothing: "*nada de cuidado* (don't work at all), for-
get about it."

The second dimension, mode of use, came across in labeling of barrier
methods like diaphragm, sponge, condom, and spermicides: "things you put
in vagina, inserted inside, have to use before sex, have to use every time";

labeling of oral contraceptive pills: "have to take it every day, *todos los días* (every day)"; and labeling of traditional methods: "you have to have trust in him, unpredictable, need control."

The third dimension was how familiar the teens themselves were with the method. All the teens who completed this task had already had the post-partum contraceptive education session in which they were taught about the various methods offered at the clinic (pills, condoms, diaphragms, spermicides, intrauterine devices, sterilization). The sixteen methods on the cards, however, included some that were not available at the clinic at the time (NORPLANT, natural family planning); one, Depo-Provera injection, that was not then available in the United States for use as a method of contraception but was easily obtained in Mexico; and several traditional methods (abstinence, rhythm, and withdrawal). In general, the least known methods were natural family planning, rhythm, and NORPLANT. If a teen did not know about a method, it was explained to her after she finished the sorting task, taking advantage of a serendipitous educational opportunity.

The fourth dimension was acceptability for personal use at this time in their lives: "these I would (or have) used, these I might use some day, and these I wouldn't use." With respect to the barrier methods, however, a significant amount of affect was apparent in labels such as "messy," "yucky," "icky," or "*los que nunca usaré* (those I will never use)," and "¡*éstos, no!* (these, no!)."

The teen mothers were also asked to rank the methods in the order in which they would actually choose to use them. Many teens ranked a subset of preferred methods, first keeping aside those that they said they would not use. After this first ranking, they were instructed to pretend that their preferred methods did not exist and to rank the remaining methods in the most acceptable order.

The mean rank for each method is given in Table 8.4. The top-ranked methods included one medical method, oral contraceptive pills, ranked first by 24% of the sample, and one barrier method, condoms, which were ranked first by 21% of the sample. Not surprisingly, these were the methods most frequently chosen by the teen mothers attending the clinic.

The second tier included NORPLANT and spermicidal foam. The appeal of NORPLANT, which was ranked first by 21% of the teens, seems to be its ease of use and length of protection. It is a coitus-independent method, and like the intrauterine device, once inserted requires no action by the user. Thus, its theoretical and typical failure rates are close to identical. None of the teens ranked any of the spermicides (cream, jelly, foam, suppositories) as their first choice. The rather high ranking of foam is probably due to its

Table 8.4.      Mean Rank Order of Use for Sixteen Methods of Contraception

| Method | N | Mean | s | Range | % | Rank 1 |
|---|---|---|---|---|---|---|
| Tier One | | | | | | |
| Oral contraceptive pill | 28 | 3.4 | 2.5 | 1–10 | 24 | |
| Condom | 28 | 3.4 | 2.6 | 1–11 | 21 | |
| Tier Two | | | | | | |
| NORPLANT | 23 | 5.5 | 4.7 | 1–16 | 21 | |
| Foam | 26 | 6.8 | 3.6 | 2–14 | 0 | |
| Tier Three | | | | | | |
| Sponge | 25 | 7.9 | 4.1 | 2–15 | 0 | |
| Depo-Provera | 25 | 8.0 | 4.5 | 1–16 | 7 | |
| Withdrawal | 25 | 8.2 | 4.1 | 1–15 | 3 | |
| Cream/jelly | 25 | 8.4 | 3.4 | 3–14 | 0 | |
| Intrauterine device | 26 | 8.5 | 4.2 | 1–16 | 3 | |
| Abstinence | 23 | 8.7 | 5.2 | 1–16 | 14 | |
| Suppositories | 24 | 8.8 | 3.3 | 4–14 | 0 | |
| Tier Four | | | | | | |
| Diaphragm | 22 | 9.2 | 3.6 | 3–16 | 0 | |
| Natural family planning | 23 | 9.4 | 5.0 | 1–16 | 7 | |
| Rhythm | 26 | 9.7 | 4.8 | 2–16 | 0 | |
| Sterilization | 23 | 10.0 | 4.5 | 2–16 | 0 | |
| No method | 25 | 11.6 | 4.0 | 4–15 | 0 | |

s = standard deviation

close association with condoms (i.e., from educational sessions in the clinic setting and their distribution together).

The third tier included a range of methods. Abstinence, which was ranked number one by 14% of the sample, is included in this tier. The intermediate ranking of withdrawal suggests that it is a method with which the teens are familiar.

The final tier also included a range of methods. Sterilization is ranked low because the young women did not feel it was appropriate for them at this time in their lives. Many actually said they would use it when they were ready to end childbearing, but not at the present time. The low ranking of the diaphragm is probably related to its mode of use, requiring a rather extensive handling of one's own genitals. Natural family planning and rhythm, which were thought to be quite similar by these young women, were also in this last group, as was the use of no method at all.

In summary, these data suggest that providers primarily view the methods they prescribe in terms of efficacy, and they tend to see medical methods as the most effective. The providers all know the theoretical and typical failure rates of the methods presented in Table 8.2 and have first-hand experience on a daily basis with pregnancies resulting from method failure or non-use. The teens, on the other hand, while using efficacy as one dimension for classifying, do not have this as their primary consideration. Rather, it is one of many factors—including mode of use and whether they like, or trust, the method enough to use it themselves—to be considered in choosing a contraceptive method.

This is, perhaps, not a surprising finding, but one about which the providers were not consciously aware. The nurse practitioners who prescribe the methods, in particular, were surprised at the results. They often had the "aha" response, "oh, so that's why . . ." As one nurse practitioner noted, "They really don't think about methods the same way we do . . . they don't think about it as just getting the most effective one." In looking at the multidimensional scaling plots and hearing what the teens said about birth control methods, they realized that teens might not always be interested in the most effective method (i.e., medical methods); rather, they utilized a number of other criteria to make their choice. The providers, on the other hand, see their job as prescribing the most effective method medically possible for the client, because they are committed to prevention of unintended pregnancy and know only too well the problems associated with the less effective (i.e., barrier) methods in this population. Moreover, many of them reflected on some of the methods they had relegated in their minds to the ineffective category (e.g., withdrawal, rhythm, etc.) but which actually have failure rates similar to the typical rates for barrier methods, and were viewed favorably by the teens. One of the nurse practitioners said, "You know, I never think of withdrawal as a birth control method, but actually it works pretty well—better than nothing—maybe I should tell them [the clients]." Another provider said:

> If we're honest, we've probably all used a combination of withdrawal and rhythm sometimes—like I calculate where I am in my cycle or if I have my period—and then I think, well, the odds are really low so I won't use anything this time. . . . Maybe we should put more effort into explaining the menstrual cycle so they [the teens] could get the "safe" time right.

While not actually able to advocate counseling teen clients to use these natural methods of birth control, providers did say they would discuss them as means of preventing pregnancy that are far better than using nothing at all but not as good as medical methods. In short, the providers gained a different perspective from which to view their clients, as more like themselves, a perspective that makes more understandable the perceived inconsistencies in their teen clients' contraceptive patterns.

Better understanding of the medical and clinic barriers to contraceptive use and teens' attitudes toward different methods available are important, but they are only part of the explanation for method noncompliance. There are also social constraints on contraceptive use by these young mothers.

## Social Constraints on Contraceptive Use

The social reasons for nonuse or discontinuation of use of contraceptive methods included relationship instability and cultural constraints on contraceptive use. The first factor identified by the TOWs, disruption of the sexual relationship with the partner, is partially a reflection of the young age of these teens, the socioeconomic circumstances in which their lives are embedded, and, probably, their stage of cognitive development (although this aspect was not formally addressed in this study). The highs and lows of adolescent emotional attachment are much greater than among older persons with more experience in interpersonal relationships. Thus, disagreements between partners may seem more serious, and break-ups that are likely to be only temporary may be perceived as permanent. Blanca notes:

> I tell them, you have a fight and he leaves—maybe he's gone a week or a month, but he'll come back. If you stop taking your pill and he comes back and the fireworks start and it's the 4th of July, then you have no protection. I tell them to be prepared—sex is good, it's OK, but they don't want another baby right away.

Moreover, many of the partners of these young women are transient themselves and migrate both within the United States and back to their countries of origin to find work or attend to family responsibilities. Any disruption in the relationship, combined with the fear of the method's effects on health status, might make discontinuation more likely.

On a different note, pregnancy is sometimes used as a test of love and commitment. Leticia's case is instructive.

*Leticia, pregnancy to test a relationship*
Leticia was 17 years old when she was first interviewed in January 1990 after giving birth to her first child, a boy. She considers herself Mexican American, has been in the United States fifteen years, and is bilingual. She had already dropped out of school before she became pregnant. At the time of delivery she lived with both her parents and seven siblings. Her family supports her economically. The baby's father, Ray, is 19 years old. He was her boyfriend, but they broke up before the baby's birth. Leticia and Ray had both wanted this pregnancy. She said she wants more children but didn't want the next one for about five years. Leticia had never used any birth control and, in fact, said she did not know there was "anything you could do."

At her postpartum appointment in February she received oral contraceptive pills. At her visit, she had a black eye, and the nurse practitioner was obliged to file a child abuse report because Leticia said her father had hit her. A week later, Leticia called the TOWs saying she was depressed about Ray leaving her. She was referred to an adolescent parent program but never went. In March, Leticia called again. She was still having problems with her boyfriend. A note on her chart said: "Patient needs extensive counseling" and "talked to neighbor who says Leticia is very much in love with Ray, but he won't have anything to do with her and she can't think about anything else."

In April, Leticia phoned the clinic. She was very upset about the child abuse report that had been filed. A week later she called again needing a referral for emergency food resources, since there was no food at her parents' house. This suggested a dysfunctional family situation. The next day she called again. She had stayed out all night and was afraid to go home because she thought her father would beat her again.

In mid-May Leticia called again. She had had unprotected sex with a new partner. She was afraid she might be pregnant and had symptoms that sounded like a urinary tract infection. She told the TOWs she had never used the pills or the foam and condoms she took at her first visit because she had to hide them from her parents. She wanted to begin using oral contraceptive pills now and was told she could start after she had her period.

A week later Leticia's mother called looking for her. She had run away from home. In late May, Leticia came to the clinic for a pregnancy test, which was positive. She had had unprotected sex again, this time with Ray, after her menses. She had not begun taking the pill because she wanted another pregnancy with Ray, but she did not know for sure if he was the father because she had also had unprotected sex with the new partner. At this point, she had decided to continue the pregnancy, and all attempts to contact her failed. Her file was closed as lost to follow-up.

The following February, Leticia came to the clinic for another pregnancy test, which was positive. She had aborted the previous pregnancy, and this time was sure she was pregnant with Ray's baby. She had never used the birth control methods provided at the clinic. She was referred for prenatal care.

Four months later, in June, she came back to the clinic requesting a pregnancy test, which was positive. In the intervening time she had had two abortions, one a pregnancy she thought had been Ray's, the other someone else's. Leticia was not sure what to do. She was back with Ray and she was pregnant. In July, Leticia was referred to Planned Parenthood for an abortion. Ray had refused to marry her, and she wanted to have the abortion to spite him. Besides, she indicated that he was a drug user and a drug dealer, and she didn't need a man like that in her life.

In December she came to the clinic for the last time, for a pregnancy test, which was positive. She said she was living at home, her mother was taking care of her first child, and she was in school trying to fulfill requirements for her General Educational Development (GED) certificate. She decided to continue this pregnancy, which was her fifth, but she didn't want to say who the father was. Since that visit, she has never been to the clinic again.

The loss of Leticia was a personal blow to the TOWs. She was a difficult case. All indications suggested that she was very much in love with Ray, who was a drug user and dealer. This elicited the sympathy of the staff. Over time, however, the TOWs came to believe that she was using her pregnancies to test his love for her, or perhaps to get him to make a commitment to her and marry her. The role of her second partner was never clear. She was purposely vague about him. Perhaps he was an attempt to elicit a jealous response from Ray, perhaps an attempt to find love in another relationship. Since the TOWs never learned the second man's name or anything about him, they concluded that Leticia was probably using him as a weapon in her quest to "get" Ray.

In the time that Leticia was involved in the Teen Project, she had everyone following her case. Although she would seem genuinely interested in preventing pregnancy and would accept contraceptive methods, she simply did not use them. To this day, just mentioning her name to the TOWs always evokes an emotional response. "Ay, Leticia, I remember her!" Blanca says:

> Some of these girls, you just wonder what's going on. They just don't seem quite right. I don't know what to do to get through to them about contraception. Leticia has been lost to follow-up so many times it's a joke, and every time she comes back pregnant. She's been pregnant five times in two years!

Although it is impossible to ever know the "truth" regarding Leticia's motivations, it is possible to envision several explanations for her behavior. First, it is possible that she was so enamored of Ray that she would do anything to "get him," thinking pregnancy would tie him to her. But each pregnancy pushed him farther away, not closer, and she would have an abortion. It is also possible that she herself was a drug user. This is certainly consistent with the impulsive and erratic behavior pattern, seemingly alternating between responsible and irresponsible choices. Third, her own family situation may have been abusive. Alternatively, her parents' reactions to her behavior—the beatings—might have been an attempt to reorient her life. The TOWs only have fragments of information on which to base their judgments. Her case will forever remain a haunting memory.

The final reason suggested by the TOWs for nonuse or discontinuance of a method was a significant other's objection to contraceptive use. It was often the case, when a teen resided with her own family, that her own mother had not come to terms with her daughter's sexuality. Blanca explains, "The mother comes in with the daughter for the check-up and tells me, 'She doesn't need that [birth control], she's not going to do that [have sex] any more.'" Or a teen's mother finds her pills and throws them away, as Lorinda notes:

> Ana told me her mother found her pills and threw them [away]—that's why she needs a pregnancy test now. I asked her why she didn't come back to the clinic for more and she said she just didn't think about it til [sic] Jorge got back. She's pregnant. I don't know what she's gonna do— third time.

Nor was it unusual for the teen's partner to prohibit her use of contraception, especially when they were married or in a stable union, thus forcing the risk of rapid repeat pregnancy upon the young woman. In fact, the TOWs have noted that there is quite a bit of social pressure from partner, family, and friends of teens in stable relationships for children to be rather closely spaced (one to two years apart). América explains:

> Yeah, the baby's getting older—maybe eight months old—and the mother-in-law starts saying "time to have another one so they'll be close. They can play together." Or maybe it's him—she wants to go to school, but he says, "no you're the mother of my child now." So he gets her pregnant again to sort of control her, keep her home. . . . I've seen it a lot.

This kind of social pressure can lead to gradual discontinuation of contraceptive use over time even though the teen herself may not want to become pregnant.

In summary, both structural and personal variables are implicated in contraceptive noncompliance. The structural variables, such as the kinds of methods available in the clinic, medical constraints on prescribing methods to individual teens, clinic hours, and travel difficulties, seem mundane but have a direct impact on the options available to the young mothers. The personal variables, including whether the teen has a sexual partner and the type of relationship they have, her relationship to her own parents, her physical state of health, her individual method preferences, and the method preferences of those close to her, also play a significant role in contraception.

To make matters more difficult, both the personal and structural variables can change, sometimes rapidly, over time. Methods come in and out of vogue, and sometimes methods are temporarily or permanently unavailable.[6] A provider willing to prescribe intrauterine devices for teens may relocate. Sexual relationships break up and new ones begin. In between, the teen may resist the idea that she will ever love anyone again. Cars break down, and telephones are disconnected. School and work create incredible time drains when combined with child care responsibilities. All of these affect contraceptive use.

In addition, strong cultural messages about contraception, pregnancy, and motherhood surface after the birth of the first child. When expressed by family and partner, they exerted considerable pressure on young mothers in a manner that supported closely spaced births (from the point of view of biomedicine) and the incompatibility of motherhood and other social roles such as school or work.

The barriers to contraceptive use, and hence to repeat-pregnancy prevention, among young Latina mothers are complex. Under such life conditions, perhaps it is surprising that less than one-quarter of the young mothers had a repeat pregnancy.

## CHAPTER NINE

# Implications for America's War on Teenage Pregnancy

Each teen who becomes pregnant does so within a specific social and cultural context with normative rules about what she should do, not just about the pregnancy, but about her whole life course. Once a Latina becomes pregnant, there are strong cultural pressures favoring motherhood and supporting traditional roles. These cultural responses are further embedded in the broader socioeconomic system in which the young woman lives, which also has a powerful influence, determining the options available to her.

There were four overall pathways to teen motherhood in this population, reflecting differences in acculturation, gender-role orientation, and life circumstances.

## Pathways to Motherhood

### The Housewife-Mother

The most common pattern was the housewife-mother. The teen following this pathway is married or living with her partner and is content with her role. She is a good mother and places priority on her children. She either planned her pregnancy or welcomed an accidental pregnancy that strengthened her relationship with her partner. She may have received prenatal care, but if she did not, it was not for lack of caring for herself and her baby, but rather lack of information or lack of access to prenatal care. Although she sometimes lives in a nuclear family, more often she lives in an extended-family situation and has considerable social support for her role from family, relatives, and friends. Her partner is working (or seeking work) and contributing to the economic support of the extended family. She may be using contraception to space her children, or she may be leaving conception to God or chance. She dropped out of school around seventh grade, and although she may want to return, she is not likely to do so because her child(ren) and her role as wife are her priorities. She may be either monolingual or bilingual, U.S.-born or foreign-born, but both she and her partner adhere to traditional male-female roles.

### The Ambivalent Mother

A second pattern was similar to the one described above, except that while adhering to traditional roles, the young mother is more ambivalent about them. She has lived in the United States long enough to realize that school and work are the way out of her current poverty and, therefore, understands better the middle-class goals and values of American society and wants to become part of it. She may be married or living with her partner, or they may be dating. Sometimes he has left her because of the pregnancy. She may have planned the pregnancy, but more often than not it was an accidental result of unplanned and unprotected intercourse. Once she became pregnant, however, she either perceived she had no choice except to have the baby or waited too long to have an abortion safely. She speaks English, most likely was in school when she got pregnant, and definitely wants to go back and to work, but feels that this is impossible now because she must take care of her baby and fulfill her duties as wife (if her partner is with her) and mother. She will probably try to go back to school after her baby is one or two years old, when child care becomes easier to find, or she may try night school or independent study toward a certificate of General Educational Development (GED). She feels the guilt and anguish of a mother who also wants a life of her own but realizes only too well the realities of caring for an infant under conditions of poverty. She will usually be a consistent contraceptor in order to wait for the "ideal" time to have another child.

### The High-Risk Mother

A third pattern was distinguished from the first two by its high-risk nature. Although this was the smallest group numerically, it was the most difficult with which to work. The teen representative of this group is either English-speaking or bilingual. She was either born in the United States or has lived here nearly her whole life and is fully acculturated to the *cholo* culture of East Los Angeles. She may have been in school when she became pregnant but probably was not a good student or a consistent attender. When she became pregnant, she dropped out. She is exposed to and often involved in the gang and drug cultures found in the barrio. She has probably experimented with alcohol, marijuana, and cocaine, but it is usually her partner who is more heavily drug and gang involved. She is involved by association with him, but she likes to "party" (drink and use drugs with him or be there when he does). Frequently her own family is described as dysfunctional by social workers. She may have been sexually or physically abused by family members, relatives, her own partner, or a neighbor. She is "hip" to the system.

She may see the baby as a way out of the gang/drug culture or she may essentially abandon her baby (usually to her mother or another relative) and continue in "the life." She may be HIV-positive and often has other sexually transmitted diseases. She often has difficulty using contraception because of her lifestyle.

### The Victim-Mother

A final pattern was associated with victimization, often of quite young (under 15 years old) teens. In this pattern, a teen was either raped, pressured to have sex, or had an accidental (or ultimately unwanted) pregnancy by a partner who left her to fend for herself. She was not happy about the pregnancy but did not abort. Rather, she neglected to take care of herself. In some cases she actively tried to provoke abortion by using drugs. This pattern brings to mind the concept of benign neglect first described by Scrimshaw (1984) with respect to living children, but here applied to the fetus during gestation. The woman is not consciously setting out to provoke miscarriage, but nevertheless, behaves in ways that might make this outcome more likely. This pattern was not specific to any cultural group or language preference.

Thus, there were four different overall life trajectories leading to the birth that brought the teens into the project. Teens exhibiting different patterns would probably have benefited from different intervention strategies. However, the Teen Project had only one intervention strategy, a clinic-based contraceptive-management and social-support program. The project focused on the negative aspects of adolescent motherhood. The intervention attempted to change individual behavior to bring it in line with middle-class expectations (i.e., minimum two-year birth spacing, return to school) without taking into consideration the sociocultural context in which these young women lived. As described above, for most of the teens, motherhood was not an obstacle, but a valued, frequently sought after, social role.

Thus, the young women used the project for their own ends—to space pregnancies, to get help negotiating the welfare system, to get referrals to other resources (housing, food, employment), and to take advantage of myriad other services the TOWs provided informally (giving rides, buying Avon products from a teen, distributing gifts of baby clothing, car seats, etc.). Only a handful of the teen mothers were able to fulfill the Teen Project's goal for them—to behave like middle-class teens. Even those who wanted to follow this course simply did not have the resources to do so— child care, family support for higher education, comfortable and stable living conditions. In the face of such obstacles, even the most highly motivated teens had great difficulty going back to school. There are tremendous obstacles to pregnancy prevention in the sociocultural context in which these young Latinas grow up. After beginning the Teen Project with great hopes to impact teenage childbearing in East L.A., we came to be happy with small successes.

Our experience with young mothers in the Teen Project suggests that unless and until changes in the opportunity structure can be effected, we might better evaluate the success of such programs in terms of the teens' own goals and improvements in their life circumstances. Three young women from the Teen Project who would have been considered failures by most program standards, but whom the TOWs consider successes, illustrate.

### Ana, self-sufficient, but not in our time frame

Ana was born in Texas and raised by her aunt. At age 17 she got pregnant accidentally, moved to Los Angeles with her boyfriend, and lived with his family in a household of eleven. After delivering her baby in 1990, she was visited by a TOW on the postpartum ward. Ana confided she had nowhere to live now that the baby was born. She never came for her postpartum appointment and was thought to be lost to follow-up.

A few months later Ana came back to Los Angeles and the counselor helped her get AFDC, Medi-Cal, and WIC, and she moved back in with her "in-laws" for two years, where she became the baby-sitter for all the children in the household. In 1992 she worked part-time in our clinic as a student worker while completing her GED. She was a consistent contraceptor, saying she wanted to wait until she was married before having any more children, even though her boyfriend was suspicious that she wanted to leave him because she would not have another child.

In 1992 she graduated from our project to the adult clinic, but would stop in to say "hi" whenever she had an appointment. She completed her GED in 1992, married her boyfriend in 1993, and they had a second baby in 1994. Ana now works as a receptionist in a local health center, he as a laborer, and they are economically self-sufficient. They bought a car and are in the process of buying a house. At 22, she has a high school degree, a job, a husband, and her two children.

### Rosa, rapid repeat pregnancy, but left physically abusive relationship with partner

Rosa was 15 years old when she was "stolen" from her family in Mexico by a 25-year-old man who raped her and brought her to the United States with him. She delivered her baby at our hospital and was picked up on the postpartum ward. Rosa has no family here, does not speak English, has only a fourth-grade education, and is completely dependent on her "husband." Rosa told her counselor that her husband keeps her and the baby locked in the room they rent and is very jealous, but he provides for her and the baby. The TOW's notes indicate that Rosa seemed depressed and anxious at that visit and was offered consultation with a social worker but declined.

Rosa has no phone, so follow-up was difficult after she missed her pill-refill appointment about six months after her baby was born. Two months later Rosa came to the clinic for a pregnancy test. She had several suspicious bruises on her face and arms but denied being beaten. She said her husband had thrown her pills away and she had not been able to come to the clinic for more. She began crying when she learned her pregnancy test was positive. The counselor suggested that she see the social worker, who could help her decide what to do, but she said no and took the referrals for prenatal care.

Four weeks later she came to the clinic with her child and asked for help—she had no one to turn to and she wanted to leave the man who had been beating her regularly. Rosa was taken to the social worker, who helped her get into a shelter, and we never heard from her again.

### Marta, repeat pregnancy after SAB

Marta was 16 years old when she migrated to the United States from Mexico with her common-law husband. She is now a traditional housewife and mother who stays home, cooks, and cleans house. Marta loves her husband, who she says is a good, kind man about six years older than she. He works as a laborer to support them. Our clinic saw Marta after she had a miscarriage with her first pregnancy. The pregnancy had been planned and very much wanted. Marta and her husband desperately want to begin their family and plan on having three children. Marta was a conscientious contraceptor, using oral contraceptive pills for a full year after her miscarriage because she wanted to comply with the doctor's recommendation to let her body recover so she would be more likely to have a healthy birth the next time she got pregnant. After the recommended year, she got pregnant soon after discontinuing her pills and delivered a healthy baby boy. She is now using Depo-Provera to space the next pregnancy the recommended two years. She and her husband are very happy. He is supportive of her using contraception for her health and the health of their children.

These cases suggest that program success might be defined differently. The project was having an impact on the lives of these young women. The TOWs were helping individuals to achieve their own goals, goals that were often quite different from those of our project. These less easily measured results are, perhaps, more important in the long run for the development of the self-esteem and empowerment that can result in self-sufficiency. It is certain that the counselors made a qualitative difference in the lives of some of the teens they served. They planted the seeds of knowledge, self-awareness, and self-esteem, but they rarely saw the long-term effects of their work. They only saw the shorter-term "failures" of repeat pregnancy and school drop-out.[1] These are the outcomes that researchers measure. They are desired outcomes in a life trajectory that is hard to attain.

Rather than abandoning prevention and amelioration programs because they fail to produce the results that we—health professionals, politicians, concerned citizens, social workers, parents—most want, perhaps we should redefine the criteria by which we measure success. These new measures must take into account the goals of the individuals we serve. Should we not also count as successes teens like Rosa, who have a repeat birth but leave an abusive relationship; those like Marta, who decide to follow medical advice about child spacing even though they run counter to the advice of friends and relatives because they want to give their children the best possible life they can; and those like Ana, who over a longer time frame succeed in both their own goals and in the broader goals of the program? This is true em-powerment, and its ultimate impact on young people's lives and those of their children is profound.

It seems obvious that short-term clinical interventions like the Teen Project are not likely to have a significant impact on teen childbearing in the absence of basic changes in the opportunity structure for these young women and their partners. Changing the lives of teen mothers like these is a much more complicated problem.

What are the implications of the different pathways to motherhood for program intervention? The ambivalent mother, whose core value system is traditional, is also strongly influenced by American values about educational achievement and middle-class lifestyles. She is torn between the two world-views and at the same time influenced by the larger socioeconomic system that makes access to health and education difficult for her. Does she realize her options are limited, or that the educational path will be difficult if she chooses it? Does she think that she will have to give up that sense of belong-ing in her family if she pursues higher education, like the college student (described by Flores in Chapter 2) who was treated as an outsider by her family? Is pregnancy, either consciously or subconsciously, a way of avoid-ing making this choice between education and family? Is this how culture shapes individual life trajectories?

What about the high-risk mother? Is she making a conscious, rational decision to use pregnancy as a way out of a self-destructive lifestyle? Or is pregnancy just a by-product of a risk-taking lifestyle that later comes to be understood as an "exit visa" or, alternatively, becomes part of a dysfunc-tional coping system (i.e., child abandonment, abuse, etc.)? Can young men use the same excuse (fatherhood) to get out? Where do we lay the blame for their involvement in the gang/drug lifestyle—on the individual, the fan . the neighborhood, the larger society, or all of them? How do we effect pregnancy prevention under such conditions? What kind of program would work with such hard-to-reach teens?

The victim-mother is most clearly at the mercy of the larger world around her, a world in which gender inequity and violence against women sometimes exact a heavier toll for some than for others. Because of anti-abortion values in her family and community, or because she waited too long to terminate, she has a child. But what kind of life will that child have? Even if the mother relinquishes the child to another family member to raise, she will still need to cope with the psychosocial consequences of being victimized. What kind of program can we offer to this category of teen mother?

Clearly, the Teen Project was not equipped to deal with these wider social, economic, and cultural considerations. The ambivalent mother needs support for continuing education. She needs child care, and she needs moral support from her family and community. She also needs support from her partner to delay further childbearing until her education is completed. The high-risk mother needs to make a break from her lifestyle, her neighborhood, her partner, and her friends, perhaps even her family. She needs a safe place to go. The victim-mother needs much more. She needs mental health services, and she needs justice for the crime committed against her.

In comparison to these three groups, the wife-mother who chooses or, after the fact, embraces her role appears to be blessed. She may be poor, but at least she knows that she is doing something right and highly valued and has the support of her partner, her family, and her religion. She is, in fact, at the center of the family, the *madre* (mother), *ama de casa* (mistress of the house). She may have problems (e.g., little money, a domineering partner), but her value system provides her with a worldview with which to cope with poverty and adversity—a worldview that Flores (1990) believes keeps Latinas down:

> Somewhere along the way, in our cocoon, we've been persuaded that to want nice houses in good neighborhoods, new cars, money, and "things" in general, is a sin. While the Catholic Church has played a big role in keeping us "humble and poor" . . . our own *gente* (the people around us) also criticize [those of] us who aspire to better things in life. We . . . are chastised with, "Trying to be Anglo?" . . . What is so Holy or so Chicano about living in overcrowded conditions or in perpetual poverty? (pp. 43–44)

Even the mother who is doing the right thing is caught in the wider socioeconomic system. She may be happy, but eventually she may come to

lores is talking about—the way traditional values trap
tional lifestyles and make extrication from poverty (via
ood jobs) seem to be a rejection of Latino culture, when it is
of class. But class and culture (i.e., race, ethnicity) have be-
twined in America today, that it is difficult to separate them.

nglo," as Flores (1990) noted, is perceived as being "middle
conflation of class and ethnicity gives rise to such epithets as
"coconut" (i.e., brown on the outside, white on the inside) for Latinos who
integrate into Anglo society and achieve socioeconomic success. This is powerful social control from a young teen's point of view. Climb out of poverty
and risk rejection. This is how culture perpetuates itself, by ostracizing those
who fail to or refuse to follow the norms and values of the community. But
culture is not static, it is always changing. The biculturalization of upwardly
mobile Latinos is a good example of the ability to retain core cultural values
while rejecting low socioeconomic status as part of the package.

So, is teen childbearing, for Latinos or any group, a good thing or a bad
thing? Certainly, we have seen the positive aspects and underlying rationality of choices made by many of the young Latinas who entered into
motherhood. A similar case has been made for inner-city and rural African
American teen mothers. There is a new generation of sociologists and econo-
mists looking at the issue of the economic rationality of teen childbearing in
the context of poverty. However rational it may seem, and however many
short-term positive aspects it may have, adolescent childbearing is detrimental in the long run. Preventing adolescent pregnancy and, failing that,
preventing rapid repeat pregnancy are important for young women's development. However important pregnancy may be in the life of an individual
teen, and however happy and appropriate early family formation may be
within a particular culture, early motherhood puts her at a disadvantage
with respect to improving her socioeconomic status and thus perpetuates her
lower-class status. In the case of Latinas and other minority teens, additional
considerations of institutional racism cannot be overlooked, and any additional barrier (i.e., motherhood) to social improvement must be removed.
Within the current socioeconomic and political context of the United States,
teenage childbearing keeps young women down.

## Implications for Prevention Programs

How, then, should our society address the teenage pregnancy problem?
In order to understand where we need to go in prevention, we need to un-
derstand where we are now. Adolescent pregnancy prevention programs in
America are hobbled by two basic problems. The first is a lack of public con-

sensus on what should be done. The second is a focus on intervention at the individual level without the necessary structural supports at the societal level.

### Values and Programs

There are really two problems of adolescent pregnancy. One is unprotected sexual activity leading to pregnancy and abortion among middle- and upper-class teens. The other is unprotected intercourse leading to pregnancy and childbearing among poor, inner-city youth, many of whom welcome, or are at least ambivalent about, becoming a mother (Zabin and Hayward 1993). Current approaches to both of these problems are the result of a deep division in American society regarding the appropriateness of premarital sex and sexual activity during adolescence. Thus, prevention is difficult because there are irreconcilable differences over the appropriate measures to implement. There are two "camps" of opinion regarding intervention strategies, each based on quite different opinions about adolescent sexual behavior.

One camp feels that premarital sexual intercourse, especially among the young, is unacceptable and immoral. They propose teaching traditional values, particularly premarital chastity, and think that other methods of prevention (e.g., contraception and abortion) have the effect of "legitimizing" and increasing premarital sexual activity. They tend to think there is too much emphasis on sex in our society and oppose the casual representation of sex in the media. Thus, the solution they offer is premarital chastity, and they disdain more liberal solutions. Within this camp, those who are most conservative also tend to oppose abortion, and the most extreme oppose contraception (Luker 1984).

The second camp is more pragmatic and, while few would advocate or promote sex among young people, they recognize that there is a large group of sexually active adolescents. This camp supports providing early education about contraception and reproduction so young people can make informed decisions. They advocate unrestricted availability of contraceptive services for adolescents and tend also to recognize the need for personal choice about abortion. They tend to be more liberal in their views about abortion and contraception, although there is considerable individual variation.

Once a young woman becomes pregnant and decides to continue the pregnancy, however, the reactions of the two groups become more similar, and both tend to favor ameliorative programs that promote a healthy birth (e.g., facilitating prenatal and other medical care). After the birth, a split again occurs, with the more conservative group favoring marriage or adoption. The second camp tends to support the decision of the young woman to relinquish or keep her child. In the latter case, they support comprehensive programs that stress school return, employment skills, and parenting classes to ameliorate the often adverse consequences of teenage childbearing.

These characterizations are a simplification of the very complicated socio-political, cultural, and ethical positions of individuals. There are variations within both groups, especially regarding how strongly the most polar positions are held. However, this is a useful framework within which to understand the relatively ineffective social response to the teenage pregnancy problem in the United States thus far.

Other industrialized countries (such as Sweden, the Netherlands, and the United Kingdom) have kept adolescent birth and abortion rates low despite high levels of sexual activity among their youth. They are straightforward in teaching young people about sex and have national policies and programs that promote responsible sexual behavior among youth. While information and access regarding contraception are important in prevention, it is really motivation to prevent pregnancy that is key. In Scandinavian countries, where levels of sexual activity among adolescents are similar to or greater than those in the United States, for example, it is not considered socially acceptable for sexually active teens to risk pregnancy by being contraceptively unprepared (Jones et al. 1985). Childbearing norms are clear and shared. Teenage sexual activity is accepted as a normal part of life, and it is dealt with in a straightforward manner. Teenage childbearing is unacceptable, and sexually active teens use contraceptives to prevent it (Hatcher et al. 1989; Jones et al. 1985).

This research suggests the importance of social values in the production of normative behavior. Any change in behavior introduced into the community must also come to have broad community support or it will ultimately fail. At present, we do not have the luxury of social consensus about adolescent reproductive behavior, and the vast differences of opinion among American adults and among leaders who formulate social policy are not lost on young people who are forming their own values regarding sexual behavior. It is hardly surprising that adolescents who are not "supposed" to be sexually active have a difficult time being contraceptively prepared. Nor is it surprising that in communities where there are many teenage mothers who receive support and assistance from family and community, teenage childbearing persists.

In the United States, most of the funding for research and intervention programs targeted toward teenage pregnancy prevention comes either from government initiatives or private foundations. Funding priorities are dictated by the particular views of those responsible for distributing the money. Both camps influence the kinds of programs available. Government funding, in particular, responds to changes in public and political opinion about appropriate research and intervention modes. Thus, under Republicans we get abstinence and adoption programs, and under Democrats we get family planning and ameliorative programs for teen mothers. Private funding is less dependent on political pressure but is, nevertheless, also influenced by these broader values. Thus, research and intervention programs tend to reflect these opposing strategies and social views about adolescent sexual and reproductive behavior.

### Focus on the Individual

Historically, most teenage pregnancy programs have concentrated on individual-level prevention, intervention, and amelioration. The broader public health approach focuses on prevention of teen pregnancy altogether (preventing or delaying sexual intercourse among schoolchildren, promoting contraception to prevent pregnancy and STIs) or the amelioration of the negative medical and socioeconomic consequences of teenage childbearing for both mother and child (medical management of the pregnant and parturient teen to effect the healthiest pregnancy outcome possible and to address postpartum health and social needs). Thus, many interventions are clinic-based extensions of health services or school-based educational programs targeting individual behavior.

Several decades of research and evaluation of prevention programs have shown only limited impact for both primary and secondary prevention efforts (Frost et al. 1995; Furstenberg et al. 1987; Luker 1991, 1996; Polit 1989; Polit and Kahn 1985). Secondary prevention programs that attempt to ameliorate the adverse consequences of teen childbearing through intensive case management, in particular, have had only limited, short-term impact (Furstenberg 1976; Polit and Kahn 1985). This is true because of funding constraints, the challenge of sustaining individual teen mothers' involvement in programs, and the difficulty of having any impact on the life of the teen in the context of social and economic supports that are grossly inadequate to meet the needs of young mothers. The failure of current programs to have more than a limited impact on adolescent pregnancy stems from social policy that focuses on individual change and grossly underestimates the powerful social, cultural, and economic forces that favor adolescent motherhood among women of color and lower socioeconomic status.

Thus, it is not surprising that short-term clinical intervention is not sufficient to alter the life course of most teenage mothers. The difficulties of caring for a baby and attending school or working are frequently insurmountable, especially considering the economic disadvantage such young families face at the outset. These problems are compounded for recent immigrants who are at a linguistic disadvantage. Moreover, undocumented status can effectively bar a young family from any hope of full participation in American society.

### Looking Beyond Individuals

Programs that focus on individuals are important and have a definite role in prevention. Yet, we cannot expect short-term programs to overcome socioeconomic barriers that make it difficult for young women to follow the counsel such programs offer (i.e., finish school, get a good job). There is a growing trend among researchers and advocates who work in the adolescent pregnancy field to call for broad changes in the socioeconomic system in order to reduce teenage childbearing. As Luker put it: "Teenage pregnancy is less about young women and their sex lives than it is about restricted horizons and the boundaries of hope. It is about race and class and how those realities limit opportunities for young people" (1991, 83). As long as we treat teen pregnancy and motherhood as an individual problem that can be "fixed" by a program or by "right-thinking," we will fail to impact young women's lives.

Nearly every major study of the antecedents of adolescent childbearing in the United States implicates minority status and socioeconomic disadvantage. Thus, it is essential to address racism and poverty in order to reduce the teenage childbearing "problem." It is easy to criticize the system but much harder to change it. Individuals like the pioneering Michael Carrera in New York City, whose program offers real opportunity to inner-city youth, are few and far between. His message is this: If we really want to help youth, we have to treat them as if they were our own and provide them with the same opportunities our own children have (Carrera 1995). Anything short of that perpetuates the inequities that make adolescent childbearing a reasonable option.

Thus, we must work to eliminate the socioeconomic constraints that keep people in poverty while at the same time providing intervention programs aimed at individuals to help them negotiate the new system. What would such changes entail? They are simple to enumerate, difficult to effect: (1) access to good education and jobs that pay a livable wage (i.e., the elimination of poverty); (2) an end to racial discrimination; (3) access to health care; (4) access to affordable, high-quality child care; and (5) paid parental leave and job security for the first two years of an infant's life.

These five strategies have broader implications for American society. American reproductive patterns are less than optimal, from both a biological and a social point of view. Childbearing is becoming increasingly polarized at both ends of the age and socioeconomic continuum.[2] Rather than focusing solely on adolescent mothers as the problem, we should try to understand the reasons for these reproductive choices. The medical risks associated with childbearing at both extremes of the childbearing years are higher than those of the optimal years. Older women (late thirties and early forties) may even be at greater risk due to the increased likelihood of disease processes that can accompany aging (hypertension, diabetes, etc.) and complicate pregnancy. Moreover, use of expensive infertility and birthing technologies often accompanies childbearing at the end of the fertile years. Yet there is no public outcry against childbearing among older, affluent, professional women even when they are not married, Murphy Brown and Dan Quayle notwithstanding.[3]

My purpose is not to condemn childbearing at either end of the spectrum, but rather to focus attention on the social, cultural, economic, and political context that has spawned radically different childbearing strategies among such disparate socioeconomic class groups. Women pursuing professional careers may be forced into delayed childbearing because of the need to devote time, energy, and effort into career building rather than family building. Without structural supports such as quality, affordable child care; flexible work or school arrangements; and realistic maternity-leave options, delayed childbearing is the only real option middle- and working-class women have in order to improve their economic status.

At the other end of the spectrum, poor adolescents of whatever race have little to gain by delaying childbearing, because they are, for the most part, already out of the higher education loop. Childbearing at an early age simply truncates education somewhat earlier. The absence of the same structural supports (child care, flexible scheduling, and maternity-leave options) that fosters delayed childbearing among professional women, makes school return very difficult if not impossible for teen mothers. Education has long been the path out of poverty in America, but it is increasingly beyond the reach of poor women. Thus, the same constraints tend to foster childbearing at the extremes of the age spectrum but for different reasons, resulting in early childbearing among the poor and late childbearing among the affluent. This, from a medical point of view, is not optimal and from a social point of view, raises many concerns.

Rather than focusing so much time and energy on the age and marital status of childbearing women, we would do better to remedy the socioeconomic constraints that lead to these childbearing extremes. What makes adolescent childbearing problematic for society is that it so often truncates opportunity, hence socioeconomic improvement and self-sufficiency. Yet this could be overcome by the institution of social supports that would allow women to bear children during the optimal reproductive ages (18–30) and still pursue education and career opportunities.

Adolescent pregnancy and childbearing are complex problems, but they are only problems in the context of our current socioeconomic system. Our system tends to punish women for childbearing during their prime child-bearing years, forcing many to choose between children and career. The re-sult is the increasing polarization of childbearing toward young ages among the lower classes and toward older ages among the higher classes. The insti-tution of social policy that is supportive of women's development and child-rearing roles could have a significant impact on the health and welfare of our nation's children.

Someone, after all, must take care of the children. Social policy that makes children the personal economic responsibility of their mothers fosters childbearing at the polar ends of the childbearing years where most risk is incurred. A broader social policy directed toward facilitating women's de-velopment by providing structural supports during the childbearing years would go a long way toward reversing the current polarized pattern. If women were assured of child care and economic assistance while pursuing higher education and career development (a time that coincides with the op-timal childbearing years), fewer would delay childbearing to the end of the reproductive span, and more young mothers would be able to continue their education. All women, and men, need quality, reliable, affordable child care; flexible education and employment arrangements for childrearing responsi-bilities; and maternity/paternity-leave policies that provide adequate time frames, economic support, and educational or employment status security.

In order to address the important issue of teenage childbearing, we must begin to understand the context in which individual behavior occurs. We must recognize the diversity of reproductive strategies in our society today, and place them in evolutionary and historical context. We must also study the broader issues that affect not only adolescents, but all women of repro-ductive age. Social, cultural, and economic trends have an important impact on human behavior that is masked when we focus only on individual behav-ior. In order to be able to formulate effective interventions, we need to dis-cover how individual behavior is related to these broader issues and identify strategies to facilitate better health and social outcomes. Only a combined strategy that addresses both the structural and individual factors that con-tribute to childbearing at the extremes of the reproductive period will facili-tate change toward childbearing during the optimal years. And, barring draconian measures, only change in the opportunity structure for poor adolescents will provide the incentives to delay childbearing. We will not impact adolescent childbearing until we address issues of racial and gender equity and the social responsibility for the health, education, and welfare of all children in America.

In this book, I have described how culture and social context combine to support early childbearing among Latina adolescents in East L.A. I have also shown why the current types of intervention programs—targeted to individual behavior change, based on middle-class life script norms, institution based, and short-term—cannot be expected to have more than a limited impact on teenage childbearing. I used the Teen Project as an example of this kind of intervention program, documenting its limited impact and explaining this by looking at the sociocultural context in which Latina teen childbearing occurs. Without changes in social structure, individuals will not have the incentive to delay childbearing.

At the individual level, this study underscores how important it is to have an understanding of teens' motivations regarding sexual intimacy, pregnancy, marriage, love, motherhood, and contraceptive use. Without this, intervention programs will continue to be irrelevant to many young women's lives. A more holistic approach toward pregnancy prevention must take into account both individual and structural aspects. At the individual level, the devastating effects of poverty, the influence of significant others, and the cultural meaning of childbearing, contraceptive use, and gender roles are important. At the structural level, issues of access to medical care, employment, child care, educational opportunities, and racism must be addressed. Only by addressing these causal factors in combination can we create the kind of environment needed to break the cycle of poverty too often associated with adolescent childbearing in this country.

Teenage pregnancy has defied solution, perhaps because, on the surface, it seems so very simple—contraception or abstinence—but at its base it is so tremendously complex, involving the most intimate and basic human experiences, needs, feelings, desires, and emotions: sex, love, reproduction, family, religion, and values. These are, perhaps, at the core of human social existence.

Many people have asked me whether, as an anthropologist, I think it is appropriate to suggest that the pattern of early childbearing among Latina adolescents, which is perceived by many as part of a cultural worldview, should be changed. Here I agree with Flores: "What is so Holy or so Chicano about . . . living in perpetual poverty?" (1990, 44). Teenage childbearing makes perpetual poverty more likely. Most Latino parents would prefer that their daughters finish high school and get married before they have children. As Erica said: "You want me to put them [the life events] in order how it should be or how I see it around here?" Latino culture is vibrant and alive. Its warmth; its love of children and genuine respect for the elderly; its reverence for mothers and fathers; and its honesty, passion, and exuberance for life are its strengths. All these can be preserved without teenage motherhood.

# Postscript

Much has changed in the Los Angeles County medical system since 1993. The January 1994 earthquake destroyed the Pediatric Hospital, and Pediatrics was joined with Women's Hospital to form Women's and Children's Hospital shortly thereafter. The family planning clinic moved across the street into the basement of a temporary out-patient building to make more room in the hospital. In 1995 it moved twice again, once after an aftershock from the Northridge quake made the temporary facilities unsafe early in the year, and again in the spring in the wake of the massive reorganization and downsizing of the LAC health care system.

Although family planning was saved in the first round of privatization of out-patient clinics, the ultimate fate of the clinic is still undecided in January 1997. The Teen Project has survived, but as a much smaller project, because of its Teen Smart Program, funded by the California Office of Family Planning.

Blanca, who had recently been promoted to a middle-management level, was one of the casualties of the LAC downsizing. She was laid off in the fall of 1995. She had been working for my research project part-time and taking courses at a community college while working full-time at the clinic. So, in a way, the layoff gave her a reprieve. It allowed her to devote more time to school, which had become a high priority now that her own children were grown. She is pursuing her B.A. in child development and working three part-time jobs: interviewing for my NICHD project,[1] counseling in the HIV clinic at LAC-USC, and working at a residential center for pregnant teens. Ironically, her biggest problem is health insurance, since she does not qualify under any of her part-time positions. Her first grandson, Nathaniel, was born in September 1996.

América is the director of the Teen Smart Program. She is the only one of the original TOWs still working with teens in the family planning clinic. Teen Smart keeps her busy with in-clinic counseling and outreach to public housing projects in the area. She and her husband had a son in April 1993.

Now that he's almost four, she is thinking about going back to school to get her master's degree in social work. She is also interviewing part-time on my research project.

Carmen is currently working as a family planning counselor in the adult clinic. She was married in June 1993. She and her husband had a baby girl in April 1995.

Lorinda left the Teen Project in May of 1994 to work for the LAC-USC Women's Health Study, a large research project tracking HIV-positive women.

Alicia still works in the clinic as a family planning counselor. She and her husband had their third daughter in 1992 and another in 1995. Although married in a civil ceremony, she and her husband will have their "real" church wedding in February 1997.

After leaving the Teen Project in 1990, Jorge continued to work with at-risk youth in various programs throughout the county. Currently, he is in charge of programs for youth in public housing. He married, and he and his wife, a physician, have a little girl.

In 1991, I took a position teaching medical anthropology at the University of Connecticut, but continued my involvement with the Teen Project, serving as a consultant and visiting once or twice a year. In 1994, I began a new research project on Latina teen pregnancy in L.A. and was there in the spring and summer of 1995. During that time, I had the demoralizing experience of witnessing the dismantling of the primary health care system and the crackdown on illegal immigrants. What is happening in L.A. is exactly the opposite of what is needed for prevention of adolescent pregnancy and childbearing. Restricting access to health, education, and welfare services can only make things worse. I love teaching and am enjoying learning about New England, but I miss L.A. I miss the climate, the ocean, my family and friends, but most of all I miss Latino culture, California-style.

# Data-Collection Forms
# and Variables

| Form | When Used | Variables |
|------|-----------|-----------|
| 1. Postpartum Ward Survey | After delivery | Demographic<br>Prenatal<br>Baby outcomes<br>Relationship to baby's father and family<br>Fertility variables<br>Plans and goals<br>Referrals |
| 2. Postpartum Telephone Check | 2 weeks after delivery | General health of mother/baby<br>Problems<br>Appointment reminder<br>Referrals |
| 3. Postpartum Appointment | 4 weeks after delivery | Demographic<br>Contraception<br>Relationship to baby's father<br>School/work<br>Problems<br>Referrals |
| 4. Risk Assessment (AIDS, STIs) | 4 weeks after delivery | Traditional risk factors (CDC)<br>Lifestyle variables |

| Form | When Used | Variables |
|---|---|---|
| 5. Clinic Revisits | Per medical protocol for contraceptive method | Demographic<br>Contraception<br>Relationship to baby's father<br>School/work<br>Problems<br>Referrals |
| 6. Telephone Method Check | Per method | Contraception<br>Relationship to baby's father<br>Referrals |
| 7. One-year Follow-up | 12 and 24 months after entry into program | Demographic<br>Contraception<br>Pregnancy<br>School<br>Relationship to baby's father |

# Methods and Variable
# Definition for Quantitative Data

## Methods

The quantitative information is based on interviews and medical-record review. Participants are interviewed on the postpartum ward within twelve to
twenty-four hours after delivery. The interview covers demographic variables, relationship to the baby's father, school and work plans, whether the
pregnancy was intended, and past and intended contraceptive use. At each
follow-up visit, cases are interviewed about these same variables. Additional
medical information is abstracted from the medical record.

## Operationalization of Variables

### Follow-up Period

Twelve months after the date of delivery for the one-year sample and
twenty-four months for the two-year sample.

### Loss to Follow-up

A teen was considered lost to follow-up if: (1) a medical record was never
opened (i.e., she never returned to the clinic); (2) she did not return to the
clinic for three months after a scheduled appointment; (3) she could not be
contacted and did not call to make an appointment at the designated time
(i.e., for annual exam, etc.); (4) the project or medical record indicated she
moved out of the area; (5) the project or medical record indicated she was
attending another health care facility; and/or (6) for cases, she had a Data
Form 11, indicating her case had been closed for the above reasons. Thus,
there can be a grace period of three months after actual loss to follow-up.
The three-month period was chosen based on staff experience with the population. Their impression was that three months would avoid closing cases

who were only temporarily not receiving care (e.g., were visiting family in Mexico or elsewhere, migrant workers, etc.).

### Months in Program at Loss to Follow-up

Number of months from the date of delivery to the date the case was closed, as outlined above.

### Clinic Return

Documentation in the medical record of return for a postpartum visit within one month of the appointment date.

### Demographic Variables

Demographic information is based on teen's self-report in the interview or on information available in the medical record.

### Number of Clinic Visits Made

The sum of the number of clinic visits documented in the medical record during the follow-up period.

### Contraceptive Methods

*Method at postpartum:* The method the teen received as documented in the medical record by the nurse practitioner or physician.

*Method at six months:* The method the teen received at the last clinic visit closest to the six-month follow-up date for teens still in the program at that time.

*Method at twelve months:* The method the teen received at the last clinic visit closest to the twelve-month follow-up date if she was not lost to follow-up at six months.

*Method at eighteen months:* The method the teen received at the last clinic visit closest to the eighteen-month follow-up date for teens still in the program at that time.

*Method at twenty-four months:* The method the teen received at the last clinic visit closest to the twenty-four-month follow-up date if she was not lost to follow-up at twelve months.

*Note:* For all contraceptive variables the categories of "none" or "missing" usually indicated that a teen had a medical problem for which she was under treatment, and was temporarily abstinent. As a part of clinic protocol, each patient was routinely given foam and condoms when she had no other method. This routine dispensing of foam and condoms is not reflected in the variable. Only when foam and condoms are the preferred/chosen method are they counted for the purposes of this follow-up.

### Repeat Pregnancy

This variable is based on verification of a positive pregnancy test documented in the patient's medical record from one–six months, six–twelve months, twelve–eighteen months, and eighteen–twenty-four months postpartum.

*Note:* Pregnancy outcome is based on the teen's personal statement about her intended resolution of the pregnancy.

### School Return

Information on this variable is based on personal report from cases in the program and was generally not available for controls.

# Notes

## Chapter 1

1. "Latino/a," a term widely used in the Southwest, will be used in this book to identify persons of Hispanic origin or ancestry from Mexico, Central America, the Caribbean, and South America, following Hurtado et al. (1992) and Molina and Aguirre-Molina (1994). Since it is a Spanish word, it has a masculine (Latino) and a feminine (Latina) form. I use Latino(s) as a noun or adjective referring to both males and females, Latina(s) when referring only to females.

2. Formerly Women's Hospital, it became Women's and Children's Hospital after the January 1994 Northridge earthquake destroyed the pediatric hospital and the two were combined under the new name.

3. *Noncompliance* is a term used in clinical care to indicate that a patient did not use or misused a drug or device prescribed for medical care.

4. At that time, in the late 1980s, drug therapy had not yet progressed to the point where we could begin to think of HIV/AIDS as a chronic, manageable disease as is the case today with the addition of protease inhibitors to the anti-HIV arsenal.

## Chapter 2

1. While the link to minority status among African Americans is predominantly through socioeconomic status, this has not yet been established definitively for Latinos in the United States, although there is little reason to suspect this relationship would not also hold among Latinos. Cooksey (1990) has demonstrated a relationship between higher parental education and use of abortion to resolve adolescent pregnancy among Latinos, although the size of the Latino subgroup was small. This is consistent with a socioeconomic effect on teenage childbearing among Latinos.

2. 200% of poverty was $23,222 for a family of four in 1988.

3. See Luker (1996) for a particularly insightful account of changes in family structure and resulting reproductive patterns.

4. Although I use the term *culture* in a manner that makes it seem like an entity in and of itself, culture is not a monolithic, static thing. Rather it is a useful heuristic device indicating a historically situated constellation of beliefs, attitudes, and behaviors that characterize a defined group or society at a point in time. Culture changes as individual behavior changes in response to new historical circumstances.

## Chapter 3

1. When the Pediatric Hospital was combined with the Women's Hospital after the 1994 Northridge earthquake destroyed the former, the number of beds for Obstetrics and Gynecology was reduced to accommodate pediatric patients.

2. Los Angeles County has an estimated metropolitan population of eight to ten million and is said to be the largest Mexican city outside of Mexico.

3. In the wake of the 1994 earthquake, the family planning clinic was relocated to temporary quarters across the street from the hospital, where it remained until an aftershock in 1995 made that building unsafe. The clinic was relocated twice again in 1995. As a result of the county's extreme budget problems in 1995, the clinic was downsized, and negotiations are currently under way to privatize the clinic.

4. This policy changed in 1994 after Proposition 187 passed. The new policy required proof of legal residence for all nonemergency services.

5. The majority of these primary health centers were privatized in 1995 following the county's budget crisis and are no longer part of the LAC system.

6. Dr. Gerald S. Bernstein, the medical director of the family planning clinic until 1995, was the principal investigator.

7. A subsequent project was funded by The William and Flora Hewlett Foundation in 1992 and ended in 1995. This project concentrated on contraceptive compliance, method type, and repeat pregnancy among teen mothers. I was a consultant on this project after leaving Los Angeles in September 1991 to take my current position at the University of Connecticut. Currently the project is funded through the Teen Smart initiative of the Office of Family Planning, State of California, and provides risk assessment and extended contraceptive counseling. In-kind support (i.e., space and clinical staff) is provided by LAC.

8. The study was funded by a grant from the University of Connecticut Research Foundation.

## Chapter 4

1. Rodney King, an African American man, was pulled over by the police while driving and was severely beaten by the officers. The event was captured on videotape by a bystander. The police officers went to trial but were acquitted. Severe rioting, looting, and arson broke out almost immediately after the verdict was handed down. Over thirty-five people were killed and millions of dollars in damage done. Curfews were imposed, schools closed, and the National Guard was called in to restore order.

2. Although extremely complex, the 1995 LAC budget crisis that resulted in the partial dismantling of the LAC health care system was due at least in part to provision of health care to the millions of indigent patients in LAC.

3. Immigrants arriving in the United States after 1981 did not qualify for amnesty under the Immigration Reform and Control Act.

4. As noted previously, the pediatric hospital was destroyed in the 1994 earthquake, and Women's Hospital became Women's and Children's Hospital. I use the name and describe the hospital and clinic as they were when the project took place.

5. In 1995 there was a Latina physician, and in 1996, the medical director was an African American woman. The current medical director as of January 1997 is Anglo.

6. RU486 is an abortifacient drug popularly known as the French abortion pill.

NORPLANT is a subdermal hormonal implant providing contraceptive protection for five years.

7. HIV is the abbreviation commonly used for the human immunodeficiency virus believed to cause the disease acquired immunodeficiency syndrome, also known as AIDS.

8. The Hewlett grant was a three-year grant with no guarantee of job stability at the end of the granting period.

## Chapter 5

1. Two hundred forty-seven Latina teen mothers were recruited as project cases between April 1989 and December 1990. This cutoff date was selected to provide a minimum of one year of follow-up for cases. Eight percent ($N = 20$) of the teens delivering during this period were not Latina and were excluded from this study. Another 22% ($N = 54$) were not interviewed on the postpartum ward and did not have the extensive background information provided by the ward survey. The larger project also included 140 controls, but their follow-up included only medical record review at twelve and twenty-four months postpartum. One hundred control subjects were interviewed on the ward. The other forty controls were missed because they delivered on the weekends, when project staff were not working. Although they were part of the intervention program, they have been excluded from this sample. Comparison of demographic characteristics (e.g., ethnicity, country of birth, reproductive history) suggests they were no different from the teens included in this study.

2. Due to constraints on staff time, ward surveys were not implemented with teen mothers who delivered at the hospital but were not returning to the family planning clinic for postpartum care during the 1989–1991 Hewlett Project. About 35% of teens in our target age group (under 18) who delivered at the hospital received appointments for postpartum care at our clinic.

3. California's Latino population has changed from being largely U.S.-born (80%) as recently as the 1960s to being largely foreign-born (65%) in the 1990s (Hurtado et al. 1992).

4. A common characteristic of multidimensional acculturation scales is the primacy of language use and preference as a measure of acculturation. Marin et al. (1987) have shown that an acculturation scale based exclusively on indicators of language use produced reliability and validity coefficients almost identical to a scale developed from a much broader range of indicators. That language is a good proxy for acculturation level was also shown by Scrimshaw et al. (1987) in a study that used an extensive acculturation scale for Mexican-origin/descent women. It also makes anthropological sense in that language is often thought of as the manner in which behavior is encoded, patterned, and expressed. Although I use the word "acculturation," a more accurate term would be "biculturation," since even the most Anglicized teens identify with Latino culture.

5. The sample is heavily weighted toward Mexican ethnicity, and the results reflect the dominance of the contribution of Mexican teens.

6. Central America is considered as one cultural area throughout this book, although there are distinct cultural and historical differences by country. In addition, most of the Central American teens in the study were from El Salvador.

7. To reduce bias in reporting, teens were asked "Was this baby planned?" and

then read the following responses: (a) yes; (b) no, but we wanted a baby at some point; (c) no, but once I knew I was pregnant I wanted the child; (d) no, I did not want to get pregnant but will keep the baby; and (e) no, I did not want to get pregnant and will give the baby up for adoption. In Table 5.3, "yes" represents all those choosing (a), "no/ok" represents all those choosing (b) or (c), and "no" represents all those choosing (d) or (e). This question had been extensively pretested in a previous study of birth among Mexican-origin women in Los Angeles and was shown to be effective in eliciting unplanned-but-wanted pregnancy as well as unwanted pregnancy (Erickson 1988; Scrimshaw, personal communication, 1986).

8. For several months the TOWs were doing an HIV risk assessment with all teens at their postpartum clinic visits. It was during these risk assessments that this type of information was divulged.

9. Multidimensional scaling is often used as an exploratory data-analysis technique because it allows the researcher to uncover "hidden structure" in the data, based on his/her knowledge of the subject or culture under study.

## Chapter 6

1. During the first year of the study, Los Angeles was experiencing a crisis within the county health system with respect to prenatal care. Demand simply outstripped supply, and waits for appointments were sometimes as long as two to four months.

2. The regression analysis included age, education level, partner support, and pregnancy intendedness as independent variables, and adequacy of care (good, intermediate, inadequate) as the dependent variable ($N = 200$).

3. In the regression, a more complicated seven-value variable of adequacy of prenatal care was used, as follows: first trimester and more than eight visits = 1; second trimester and more than three visits = 2; third trimester and more than three visits = 3; first trimester and fewer than eight visits = 4; second trimester and fewer than four visits = 5; third trimester and fewer than four visits = 6; and no care = 7.

## Chapter 7

1. The control group was no different from the case group regarding language and cultural group. As indicated in Chapter 2, however, the controls may have been a slightly lower-risk group because TOWs were allowed to shift high-risk teens from control status to case status.

2. Foam and condoms, although two separate contraceptive methods, are treated as a single method in the clinic.

3. Number of children desired was estimated by adding parity and number of additional children desired for the 127 teens who provided a definite response to the question.

4. The three cultural groups were compared using SAS General Linear Models, with length of time in the program as the dependent variable and cultural group as the independent variable.

5. There had been no studies of retention in care for this population group. Our estimates were based on the "best guess" consensus of the health care providers and on the rate for failed appointments, which was about 50% for the postpartum visit.

6. The following section on the factors contributing to loss of follow-up (pp. 124–126) is reproduced with the permission of The Alan Guttmacher Institute from "Lessons from a Repeat Pregnancy Prevention Program for Hispanic Teenage Mothers in East Los Angeles" (Erickson 1994a, 174–178).

7. Among the controls, the one-year repeat-pregnancy rate was 18%, but the size of the sample after loss to follow-up was too small to draw valid quantitative comparisons.

### Chapter 8

1. This was addressed in the second Hewlett Project, which tracked contraceptive method compliance and repeat pregnancy.

2. This study was undertaken before Depo-Provera and NORPLANT became available to clinic clients in 1992.

3. Portions of the sections "Factors Affecting Contraceptive Use" and "Medical Methods" (pp. 133–137) are reproduced with the permission of The Alan Guttmacher Institute from "Lessons from a Repeat Pregnancy Prevention Program for Hispanic Teenage Mothers in East Los Angeles" (Erickson 1994a, 174–178).

4. The addition in 1992 of Depo-Provera and NORPLANT to the contraceptive methods offered at the clinic helped to remedy some of the problems associated with the other methods. NORPLANT, a five-year contraceptive implant, seems to be less used than Depo-Provera, a three-month injection. Neither method is coitus dependent nor necessitates daily effort on the part of the user.

5. The results of this study have been published previously (Erickson 1996).

6. For example, intrauterine devices were temporarily unavailable to U.S. women in the late 1980s after lawsuits brought against the makers of the Dalkon Shield forced other IUDs off the market. Depo-Provera, which was widely used throughout the world for many years, was not approved by the U.S. Food and Drug Administration for use as a contraceptive in the United States until 1992.

### Chapter 9

1. The only really long-term follow-up of adolescent mothers suggests that ameliorative programs do have a significant effect on life circumstances seventeen years later. It is interesting to note that this same study did not find significant effects at five-year follow-up when the young mothers were typically doing least well. This suggests that the influence of programs and services may not be detectable during the shorter term, and that a much longer perspective than is generally feasible in research designs is needed to fully understand ultimate program impact (Furstenberg 1987).

2. See Luker (1996) for a fuller development of this theme.

3. *Murphy Brown* is a popular television show about a mature woman who is a successful career TV newswoman. In real life, the actress Candace Bergen became pregnant. For the duration of her pregnancy, the plot followed her from her decision to become an unwed mother through the difficulties of being a single parent even under affluent circumstances. Then–Vice President Dan Quayle castigated the show for promoting unwed motherhood.

## Postscript

1. This five-year project is funded by the National Institute for Child Health and Development (R29HD32351) and includes collection of life histories from fifty teen mothers, their partners, and nonmother "controls" and collection of survey data from one thousand Latina teen mothers operationalizing life themes from the life history data.

# Bibliography

Alvirez, D. 1973. The Effects of Formal Church Affiliation and Religiosity on the Fertility Patterns of Mexican American Catholics. *Demography* 10: 19–36.

Amaro, Hortensia. 1988. Women in the Mexican-American Community: Religion, Culture, and Reproductive Attitudes and Experiences. *Journal of Community Psychology* 16: 6–20.

Andolsek, Kathryn M. 1990. *Obstetric Care: Standards of Prenatal, Intrapartum and Postpartum Management.* Philadelphia: Lea & Febiger.

Andrade, Sally S. 1980. Family Planning Practices of Mexican Americans. In *Twice a Minority,* ed. Margarita Melville. St. Louis: C. V. Mosby, 17–32.

Aneshensel, Carol S., Eve Fielder, and Rosina M. Becerra. 1989. Fertility and Fertility-related Behavior among Mexican-American and Non-Hispanic White Female Adolescents. *Journal of Health and Social Behavior* 30 (March): 56–76.

Baird, Traci L. 1993. Mexican Adolescent Sexuality: Attitudes, Knowledge, and Sources of Information. *Hispanic Journal of Behavioral Sciences* 15(3): 402–417.

Balcazar, Héctor, and Carolyn Aoyama. 1991. Interpretive Views of Hispanics' Perinatal Problems of Low Birth Weight and Prenatal Care. *Public Health Reports* 106(4): 420–426.

Baldwin, Wendy, and Virginia S. Cain. 1980. The Children of Teenage Parents. *Family Planning Perspectives* 12(1): 34–43.

Barret, Robert L., and Bryan E. Robinson. 1982a. A Descriptive Study of Teenage Expectant Fathers. *Family Relations* 31 (July): 349–352.

———. 1982b. Teenage Fathers: Neglected Too Long. *Social Work* 27(6): 484–488.

Bean, Frank D., and Marta Tienda. 1987. *The Hispanic Population of the United States.* New York: Russell Sage Foundation.

Becerra, Rosina M., and Diane de Anda. 1984. Pregnancy and Motherhood among Mexican American Adolescents. *Health and Social Work* 9(2): 106–123.

Bello, Teresa A. 1979. The Latino Adolescent. In *Perspectives on Adolescent Health Care,* ed. Ramona T. Mercer. St. Louis: C. V. Mosby, 57–64.

Berenson, Abbey B., Virginia V. San Miguel, and Gregg S. Wilkinson. 1992. Prevalence of Physical and Sexual Assault in Pregnant Adolescents. *Journal of Adolescent Health* 13(6): 466–469.

Berlin, Cydelle, and Laura Berman. 1994. The Other Partner. *Family Life Educator* 12(3): 4–10.

Bernard, H. Russell. 1994. *Research Methods in Anthropology.* 2d ed. Thousand Oaks, Calif.: Sage Publications.

Blum, Roger W. 1991. Global Trends in Adolescent Health. *Journal of the American Medical Association* 265(20): 2711–2719.

Bongaarts, John. 1982. The Fertility Inhibiting Effects of the Intermediate Fertility Variables. *Studies in Family Planning* 13(6/7): 179–189.

Boone, Margaret S. 1988. Social Support for Pregnancy and Childbearing Among Disadvantaged Blacks in an American Inner City. In *Childbirth in America: Anthropological Perspectives,* ed. Karen L. Michaelson and Contributors. South Hadley, Mass.: Bergin & Garvey Publishers, 66–78.

Borgatti, Stephen P. 1992. *ANTHROPAC 4.04.* Columbia, S.C.: Analytic Technologies.

Boyer, Debra, and David Fine. 1992. Sexual Abuse as a Factor in Adolescent Pregnancy and Child Maltreatment. *Family Planning Perspectives* 24(1): 4–11, 19.

Braverman, Paula K., and Victor C. Strasburger. 1993. Adolescent Sexual Activity. *Clinical Pediatrics* 32(11): 658–668.

Brindis, Claire D., and Rita J. Jeremy. 1988. *Adolescent Pregnancy and Childbearing in California: Building a Strategic Plan for Action.* San Francisco: Center for Population and Reproductive Health Policy Studies, UCSF.

Brown, Sarah S., ed. 1988. *Prenatal Care: Reaching Mothers, Reaching Infants.* Institute of Medicine. Washington, D.C.: National Academy Press.

Burt, Martha R. 1986. *Estimates of Public Costs for Teenage Childbearing.* Washington, D.C.: Center for Population Options.

Burton, Linda M. 1990. Teenage Childbearing as an Alternative Life Course Strategy in Multigeneration Black Families. *Human Nature* 1(2): 123–143.

Card, Josephina J. 1981. Long-term Consequences for Children of Teenage Parents. *Demography* 18(2): 137–156.

Card, Josephina J., and L. Wise. 1978. Teenage Mothers and Teenage Fathers: The Impact of Early Childbearing on the Parents' Personal and Professional Lives. *Family Planning Perspectives* 10: 199–205.

Carerra, Michael. 1995. "Teen Sexuality: Realistic Approaches, Positive Messages." Keynote address given at plenary session, 15th anniversary conference, Advocates for Youth, Washington, D.C., December 8–10.

Center for Population Options. 1989. "Teenage Pregnancy and Too-Early Childbearing: Public Costs, Personal Consequences." Washington, D.C.: Center for Population Options.

Chinchilla, Norma, Nora Hamilton, and James Loucky. 1993. Central Americans in Los Angeles: An Immigrant Community in Transition. In *In the Barrios. Latinos and the Underclass Debate,* ed. Joan Moore and Raquel Pinderhughes. New York: Russell Sage Foundation, 51–78.

Christopher, F. Scott, Diane C. Johnson, and Mark W. Roosa. 1993. Family, Individual, and Social Correlates of Early Hispanic Adolescent Sexual Expression. *The Journal of Sex Research* 30(1): 54–61.

Conover, Ted. 1987. *Coyotes: A Journey Through the Secret World of America's Illegal Aliens.* New York: Vintage Departures.

Cooksey, Elizabeth C. 1990. Factors in the Resolution of Adolescent Pregnancy. *Demography* 27(2): 207–218.

Cousineau, Michael R. 1995. Who Can Pay? Who Will Pay? *UCLA Magazine* 7(3): 24.

Darabi, Katherine F., Joy Dryfoos, and Dana Schwartz. 1986. Hispanic Adolescent Fertility. *Hispanic Journal of Behavioral Sciences* 8(2): 157–171.

Darabi, Katherine F., Elizabeth H. Graham, and Susan G. Philliber. 1982. The Second Time Around: Birth and Birth Spacing among Teenage Mothers. Chap. 19 in *Pregnancy in Adolescence*, ed. Irving R. Stuart and Carl F. Wells. New York: Van Nostrand, 427–437.

Darabi, Katherine F., and Vilma Ortiz. 1987. Childbearing among Young Latino Women in the United States. *American Journal of Public Health* 77(1): 25–28.

Davis, Kingsley. 1980. A Theory of Teenage Pregnancy in the United States. Chap. 12 in *Adolescent Pregnancy and Childbearing*, ed. Catherine S. Chilman. Washington, D.C.: U.S. Dept. of Health and Human Services, Public Health Service, National Institutes of Health, 309–339.

Davis, Kingsley, and Judith Blake. 1956. Social Structure and Fertility. *Economic Development and Social Change* 4(4): 211–235.

Dryfoos, Joy. 1982. The Epidemiology of Adolescent Pregnancy: Incidence, Outcomes, and Interventions. In *Pregnancy in Adolescence. Needs, Problems, and Management*, ed. Irving R. Stuart and Carl F. Wells. New York: Van Nostrand Reinhold, 27–47.

———. 1990. *Adolescents at Risk. Prevalence and Prevention.* New York: Oxford University Press.

DuRant, Robert H., Robert Pendergrast, and Carolyn Seymore. 1990. Sexual Behavior Among Hispanic Female Adolescents in the United States. *Pediatrics* 85(6): 1051–1058.

Eisenberg, Merrill R. 1984. *Teenage Childbearing in a Small New England Town: The Influence of Social, Nutritional, and Behavioral Factors.* Ph.D. diss., University of Connecticut.

Erickson, Pamela I. 1987. Sexual Attitudes and Behaviors of Minority Teens. Paper presented at the annual meeting of the American Anthropological Association, Chicago, Ill., November 18–22.

———. 1988. *Pregnancy and Childbirth among Mexican-Origin Teenagers in Los Angeles.* Ph.D. diss., University of California, Los Angeles.

———. 1990. Improving the Use of Perinatal Services among Latinas in Los Angeles County. Chap. 2 in *Task Force Report on Improving the Delivery of Health and Social Services to Latina Immigrant Women and Children in Los Angeles County.* Claremont, Calif.: Tomás Rivera Center, an affiliated institution of the Claremont Graduate School, Claremont, Calif.

———. 1994a. Lessons from a Repeat Pregnancy Prevention Program for Hispanic Teenage Mothers in East Los Angeles. *Family Planning Perspectives* 26, no. 4 (July/August): 174–178.

———. 1994b. Hispanic Women's Perspectives on Sexual Behavior and Romantic Relationships. Paper presented at the annual meeting of the American Anthropological Association, Atlanta, Ga., November 30–December 4.

———. 1996. Contraceptive Methods: Do Hispanic Adolescents and Their Family Planning Care Providers Think about Contraceptive Methods the Same Way? *Medical Anthropology* 17: 65–82.

Erickson, Pamela I., and Celia P. Kaplan. 1992. Abortion among Hispanic Women in the U.S.: Data from H-HANES. Paper presented at the annual meeting of the American Public Health Association, Washington, D.C., November 8–12.

Erickson, Pamela I., Rebecka I. Lundgren, and Anemeli Monroy de V. 1989. Comparisons of Adolescents Delivering at Public Hospitals in Mexico City and Los Angeles. Paper presented at the annual meeting of the American Public Health Association, Chicago, Ill., October 22–26.

Erickson, Pamela I., and Andrea J. Rapkin. 1991. Unwanted Sexual Experiences among Middle and High School Students. *Journal of Adolescent Health Care* 12: 319–325.

Erickson, Pamela I., Andrea J. Rapkin, Susan C. M. Scrimshaw, Thomas J. Long, Sallie J. Pappas, and Adrienne Davis. 1987. Multiple Risk-taking Behavior in Middle and High School Students in the Los Angeles Metropolitan Area. Paper presented at the annual meeting of the American Public Health Association, New Orleans, La., October 18–22.

Erickson, Pamela I., and Jorge Reyes. 1990. Case Management of High-risk Teen Mothers: Repeat Pregnancy, School Return, and the Problem of Physical and Sexual Abuse. Paper presented at the 118th annual meeting of the American Public Health Association, New York, N.Y., September 30–October 4.

Erickson, Pamela I., and Susan C. M. Scrimshaw. 1985. Contraceptive Knowledge and Intentions among Latina Teenagers Experiencing Their First Birth. Los Angeles: University of California at Los Angeles, Institute for Social Science Research, *Working Papers in the Social Sciences*, Vol. 1, no. 1.

Esparza, R. 1979. *The Value of Children among Lower-class Mexican, Mexican American, and Anglo Couples.* Ph.D. diss., University of Texas, San Antonio.

Felice, Marianne E., Paul Shragg, Michelle James, and Dorothy R. Hollingsworth. 1986. Clinical Observations of Mexican American, Caucasian, and Black Pregnant Teenagers. *Journal of Adolescent Health Care* 7: 305–310.

———. 1987. Psychosocial Aspects of Mexican-American, White, and Black Teenage Pregnancy. *Journal of Adolescent Health Care* 8: 330–335.

Fennelly, Katherine. 1993. Sexual Activity and Childbearing among Hispanic Adolescents in the United States. In *Early Adolescence: Perspectives on Research, Policy, and Intervention,* ed. Richard M. Lerner. Hillsdale, N.J.: Lawrence Eribaum Associates, 335–352.

Flores, Bettina R. 1990. *Chiquita's Cocoon: A Cinderella Complex for the Latina Woman.* Granite Bay, Calif.: Pepper Vine Press.

Ford, Clellan Stearns. 1964. *A Comparative Study of Human Reproduction.* Yale University Publications in Anthropology, no. 32. New Haven: Yale Human Relations Area Files Press.

Ford, Clellan Stearns, and Frank A. Beach. 1951. *Patterns of Sexual Behavior.* New York: Harper & Brothers.

Ford, Kathleen. 1983. Second Pregnancies among Teenage Mothers. *Family Planning Perspectives* 15(6): 268–272.

Ford, Kathleen, and Anne E. Norris. 1993. Urban Hispanic Adolescents and Young Adults: Relationship of Acculturation to Sexual Behavior. *The Journal of Sex Research* 30(4): 316–323.

Forrest, Jacqueline D. 1993. Timing of Reproductive Life Stages. *Obstetrics and Gynecology* 82(1): 105–111.

Forrest, Jacqueline D., and Susheela Singh. 1990. The Sexual and Reproductive Behavior of American Women, 1982–1988. *Family Planning Perspectives* 22(6): 206–214.

Franklin, Donna L. 1988. Race, Class, and Adolescent Pregnancy: An Ecological Analysis. *American Journal of Orthopsychiatry* 58(3): 339–354.

Frost, Jennifer J., and Jacqueline Darroch Forrest. 1995. Understanding the Impact of Effective Teenage Pregnancy Prevention Programs. *Family Planning Perspectives* 27(5): 188–195.

Furstenberg, Frank F. 1976. *Unplanned Parenthood: The Social Consequences of Teenage Childbearing.* New York: Free Press.

Furstenberg, Frank F., J. Brooks-Gunn, and S. Philip Morgan. 1987. *Adolescent Mothers in Later Life.* Cambridge: Cambridge University Press.

Geronimus, Arline T. 1991. Teenage Childbearing and Social and Reproductive Disadvantage: The Evolution of Complex Questions and the Demise of Simple Answers. *Family Relations* 40: 463–471.

Geronimus, Arline T., and Sanders Korenman. 1993. Maternal Youth or Family Background? On the Health Disadvantages of Infants with Teenage Mothers. *American Journal of Epidemiology* 137(2): 213–224.

González, Judith Teresa. 1993. Dilemmas of the High-achieving Chicana: The Double Bind Factor in Male/Female Relationships. In *Mexican American Identity,* ed. Martha E. Bernal and Phylis C. Martinelli. Encino, Calif.: Floricanto Press, 141–157.

Gordon, Sol, Peter Scales, and Kathleen Everly. 1979. *The Sexual Adolescent: Communicating with Teenagers about Sex.* 2d ed. North Scituate, Mass.: Duxbury Press.

Graham, David. 1981. The Obstetric and Neonatal Consequences of Adolescent Pregnancy. In *Pregnancy and Childbearing during Adolescence: Research Priorities for the 1980s.*(Proceedings of a conference held October 5–7 at Canandaigua, N.Y., sponsored by March of Dimes Birth Defects Foundation and University of Rochester Medical Center), ed. Elizabeth R. McAnarney and Gabriel Stickle. Birth Defects Original Article Series 17, no. 3. New York: Liss, 49–67.

Grebler, Leo, Joan W. Moore, and Ralph C. Guzman. 1970. *The Mexican American People, the Nation's Second Largest Minority.* New York: Free Press.

Alan Guttmacher Institute. 1976. *Eleven Million Teenagers: What Can Be Done about the Epidemic of Adolescent Pregnancies in the United States.* New York: Alan Guttmacher Institute.

———. 1981. *Teenage Pregnancy: The Problem That Hasn't Gone Away.* New York: Alan Guttmacher Institute.

Hardy, Janet. 1982. Adolescents as Parents: Possible Long-range Implications. In *Promoting Adolescent Health,* ed. Thomas J. Coates, et al. New York: Academic Press, 255–267.

———. 1988. Teenage Pregnancy: An American Dilemma. In *Maternal and Child Health Practices,* ed. Helen M. Wallace, George Ryan, Jr., and Allan C. Oglesby. 3d ed. Oakland, Calif.: Third Party Publishing, 539–554.

Hardy, Janet, Anne K. Duggan, Katya Masnyk, and Carol Pearson. 1989. Fathers of Children Born to Young Urban Mothers. *Family Planning Perspectives* 21(4): 159–163.

Harris, Mary G. 1988. *Cholas: Latino Girls and Gangs.* New York: AMS Press.

Hatcher, Robert A., Felicia Guest, Felicia Stewart, Gary K. Stewart, James Trussell, Sylvia Cerel Bowen, and Willard Cates. 1989. *Contraceptive Technology 1988– 1989*. 14th ed. New York: Irvington Publishers.

Hatcher, Robert A., Gary K. Stewart, Felicia Stewart, Felicia Guest, David W. Schwartz, and Stephanie A. Jones. 1981. *Contraceptive Technology 1980– 1981*. 10th rev. ed. New York: Irvington Publishers.

Hayes, Cheryl, ed. 1987. *Risking the Future: Adolescent Sexuality, Pregnancy, and Childbearing*. Volume 1. Washington, D.C.: National Academy Press.

Hayes-Bautista, David E., Werner O. Schink, and Jorge Chapa. 1988. *The Burden of Support: Young Latinos in an Aging Society*. Stanford: Stanford University Press.

Hendricks, Leo E., and Teresa Montgomery. 1983. A Limited Population of Unmarried Adolescent Fathers: A Preliminary Report of Their Views on Fatherhood and the Relationship with the Mothers of Their Children. *Adolescence* 18(69): 201–210.

Henshaw, Stanley K., and J. Silverman. 1988. The Characteristics and Prior Contraceptive Use of U.S. Abortion Patients. *Family Planning Perspectives* 20(4): 158–168.

Hotvedt, M. E. 1976. *Family Planning among Mexican Americans in South Texas*. Ph.D. diss., Indiana University.

Hurtado, Aida, David E. Hayes-Bautista, R. Burciaga Valdez, and Anthony C. R. Hernández. 1992. *Redefining California: Latino Social Engagement in a Multicultural Society*. Los Angeles: UCLA Chicano Studies Research Center.

Jacobs, Janet L. 1994. Gender, Race, Class, and the Trend toward Early Motherhood. *Journal of Contemporary Ethnography* 22(4): 442–462.

Jencks, Christopher. 1990. Is the American Underclass Growing? In *The Urban Underclass*, ed. Christopher Jencks and Paul E. Peterson. Washington, D.C.: The Brookings Institute, 28–100.

John, A. Meredith, and Reynaldo Martorell. 1989. Incidence and Duration of Breastfeeding in Mexican-American Infants, 1970–1982. *American Journal of Clinical Nutrition* 50: 868–874.

Jones, Elisa F., Jacqueline Darroch Forrest, Noreen Goldman, Stanley K. Henshaw, Richard Lincoln, Jeannie I. Rosoff, Charles F. Westoff, and Deirdre Wulf. 1985. Teenage Pregnancy in Developed Countries: Determinants and Policy Implications. *Family Planning Perspectives* 17(2): 53–62.

Jordan, Brigitte. 1978. *Birth in Four Cultures: A Cross-Cultural Investigation of Childbirth in Yucatan, Holland, Sweden, and the United States*. St. Albans, Vt.: Eden Press Women's Foundation.

Joyce, Theodore J. 1988. The Social and Economic Correlates of Pregnancy Resolution among Adolescents in New York City by Race and Ethnicity: A Multivariate Analysis. *American Journal of Public Health* 78: 626–631.

Joyce, Theodore J., and Michael Grossman. 1990. Pregnancy Wantedness and the Early Initiation of Prenatal Care. *Demography* 27(1): 1–17.

Kaplan, Celia P. 1990. *Critical Factors Affecting School Dropout among Mexican-American Women*. Ph.D. diss., University of California, Los Angeles.

Kaplan, Celia P., and Pamela I. Erickson. 1997. The Effects of Acculturation, Gender Role Orientation, and Familism on Abortion among Adolescent and Young Latinas. Article submitted to *Family Planning Perspectives*, January 1997.

Kay, Margarita A. 1978. The Mexican-American. In *Culture/Childbearing/Health Professionals*, ed. Ann L. Clark. Philadelphia: F. A. Davis, 88–108.

———. 1980. Mexican American and Chicana Childbirth. In *Twice a Minority*, ed. Margarita Melville. St. Louis: C. V. Mosby, 52–65.

———. 1982. *Anthropology of Human Birth*. Philadelphia: F. A. Davis.

Konner, Melvin, and Majorie Shostak. 1986. Adolescent Pregnancy and Childbearing: An Anthropological Perspective. In *School-Age Pregnancy and Parenthood: Biosocial Dimensions*, ed. Jane B. Lancaster and Beatrix A. Hamburg. New York: Aldine, De Gruyter, 325–346.

Kotelchuck, Milton. 1994. An Evaluation of the Kessner Adequacy of Prenatal Care Index and a Proposed Adequacy of Prenatal Care Utilization Index. *American Journal of Public Health* 84(9): 1414–1420.

Kranau, Edgar J., Vicki Green, and Gloria Valencia-Weber. 1982. Acculturation and the Hispanic Woman: Attitudes toward Women, Sex-Role Attribution, Sex-Role Behavior, and Demographics. *Hispanic Journal of Behavioral Sciences* 1: 21–40.

Kriepe, Ronald E. 1983. Prevention of Adolescent Pregnancy: A Developmental Approach. In *Premature Adolescent Pregnancy and Parenthood*, ed. Elizabeth R. McAnarney. New York: Grune and Stratton, 37–60.

Kruskall, Joseph B., and Myron Wish. 1978. *Multidimensional Scaling*. Sage University Series on Quantitative Applications in the Social Sciences, no. 07-011. Newbury Park, Calif.: SAGE Publications.

Kunitz, Stephen J. 1989. *Disease Change and the Role of Medicine: The Navajo Experience*. Berkeley: University of California Press.

Lancaster, Jane B., and Beatrix A. Hamburg, eds. 1986. *School-Age Pregnancy and Parenthood: Biosocial Dimensions*. New York: Aldine, De Gruyter.

Landry, David J., and Jacqueline Darroch Forrest. 1995. How Old Are U.S. Fathers? *Family Planning Perspectives* 27(4): 159–161.

Laumann, Edward O., John H. Gagnon, Robert T. Michael, and Stuart Michaels. 1994. *The Social Organization of Sexuality: Sexual Practices in the United States*. Chicago: University of Chicago Press.

Lazarus, Wendy, and Kathleen M. West. 1987. *Back to Basics: Improving the Health of California's Next Generation. Executive Summary*. A Report of the Children's Research Institute of California and Southern California Child Health Network. Santa Monica, Calif.: Southern California Child Health Network.

Lee, Sally Hughes, and Laurie M. Grubbs. 1994. Pregnant Teenagers' Self-Reported Reasons for Seeking or Not Seeking Prenatal Care. *Florida Nurse* 42(4): 6.

Leibowitz, A., M. Eisen, and W. K. Chow. 1986. An Economic Model of Teenage Pregnancy Decision Making. *Demography* 23: 67–79.

Leland, N. L., and R. P. Barth. 1992. Gender Differences in Knowledge, Intentions, and Behaviors Concerning Pregnancy and Sexually Transmitted Disease Prevention among Adolescents. *Journal of Adolescent Health* 13: 589–599.

Luker, Kristin. 1984. The War between the Women. *Family Planning Perspectives* 16: 105–110.

———. 1991. Dubious Conceptions: The Controversy Over Teen Pregnancy. *The American Prospect* 5: 73–83.

———. 1996. *Dubious Conceptions: The Politics of Teenage Pregnancy*. Cambridge, Mass.: Harvard University Press.

Lupton, Deborah. 1994. *Medicine as Culture: Illness, Disease, and the Body in West-ern Society.* London: SAGE Publications.

Marin, Barbara V., Gerardo Marin, and Amado M. Padilla. 1981. Attitudes and Prac-tices of Low-Income Hispanic Contraceptors. *Spanish-Speaking Mental Health Research Center,* Occasional Paper No. 13. Los Angeles: University of Califor-nia at Los Angeles.

Marin, Gerardo, Fabio Sabogal, Barbara V. Marin, Regina Otero-Sabogal, and Eliseo J. Pérez-Stable. 1987. Development of a Short Acculturation Scale for Hispanics. *Hispanic Journal of the Behavioral Sciences* 9(2): 183–205.

Marini, Margaret Mooney. 1978. The Transition to Adulthood: Sex Differences in Educational Attainment and Age at Marriage. *American Sociological Review* 43: 483–507.

———. 1984. Women's Educational Attainment and the Timing of Entry into Par-enthood. *American Sociological Review* 49: 491–511.

Markides, K., and Jeannine Coreil. 1986. The Health of Hispanics in the Southwest-ern United States: An Epidemiological Paradox. *Public Health Reports* 101: 253–265.

Marsiglio, William. 1993. Adolescent Males' Orientation toward Paternity and Con-traception. *Family Planning Perspectives* 25(1): 22–31.

Martinez, Angel Luis. 1981. The Impact of Adolescent Pregnancy on Hispanic Ado-lescents and Their Families. In *Teenage Pregnancy in a Family Context,* ed. Theodora Ooms. Philadelphia: Temple University Press, 326–343.

McElroy, Ann, and Patricia K. Townsend. 1989. *Medical Anthropology in Ecological Perspective.* 2d ed. Boulder, Col.: Westview Press.

Mead, Margaret, and Niles Newton. 1967. Cultural Patterning of Perinatal Behavior. In *Childbearing: Its Social and Psychological Aspects,* ed. Stephen A. Richard-son and Alan F. Guttmacher. Baltimore: Williams and Wilkins, 142–244.

Medina, Antonio S. 1979. Hispanic Reproductive Health in California, 1976–1977. Paper presented at Dept. of Health, Education and Welfare, Public Health Ser-vice, Hispanic Heritage Week Celebration, Rockville, Md., September 11.

Melville, Margarita B., ed. 1980. *Twice a Minority: Mexican-American Women.* St. Louis: C. V. Mosby.

Menken, Jane. 1981. The Health Consequences of Early Parenthood. In *Teenage Sexuality, Pregnancy, and Childrearing,* ed. Frank F. Furstenburg, et al. Phil-adelphia: University of Pennsylvania Press, 167–183.

Miller, Brent C., and Kristin A. Moore. 1990. Adolescent Sexual Behavior, Preg-nancy, and Parenting: Research through the 1980s. *Journal of Marriage and the Family* 52 (November): 1025–1044.

Miller, Warren B., and Lucille F. Newman, eds. 1978. *The First Child and Family Formation.* Chapel Hill: Carolina Population Center.

Mirande, Alfredo, and Evangelina Enríquez. 1979. *La Chicana: The Mexican-American Woman.* Chicago: University of Chicago Press.

MMWR (*Morbidity and Mortality Weekly Report*). 1993. Childbearing Patterns among Selected Racial/Ethnic Minority Groups—United States, 1990. *MMWR* 42, no. 20 (May 28, 1993): 398–403.

Molina, Carlos W., and Marilyn Aguirre-Molina. 1994. *Latino Health in the U.S.: A Growing Challenge.* Washington, D.C.: American Public Health Association.

Moore, Joan, and Raquel Pinderhughes, eds. 1993. *In the Barrios: Latinos and the Underclass Debate*. New York: Russell Sage Foundation.

Moore, Joan, and James Diego Vigil. 1993. Barrios in Transition. In *In the Barrios: Latinos and the Underclass Debate*, ed. Joan Moore and Raquel Pinderhughes. New York: Russell Sage Foundation, 27–49.

Moore, Kirsten A., and Martha R. Burt. 1982. *Private Crisis, Public Cost. Policy Perspectives on Teenage Childbearing*. Washington, D.C.: The Urban Institute Press.

Mosher, William D., and Christine A. Bachrach. 1987. First Premarital Contraceptive Use: United States, 1960–1982. *Studies in Family Planning* 18(2): 83–95.

Mosher, William D., and Marjorie C. Horn. 1988. First Family Planning Visit by Young Women. *Family Planning Perspectives* 20(1): 33–40.

Mosher, William D., and J. W. McNally. 1991. Contraceptive Use at First Premarital Intercourse: United States, 1965–1988. *Family Planning Perspectives* 23(3): 108–122.

Moss, Nancy, and Paul A. Hensleigh. 1991. Initiation of Prenatal Care by Adolescents: Associations with Social Support, Stress, and Hispanic Ethnicity. *Journal of Perinatology* 10(2): 170–174.

Mott, Frank L. 1986. The Pace of Repeated Childbearing among Young American Mothers. *Family Planning Perspectives* 18(1): 5–12.

Mott, Frank L., and R. Jean Huarin. 1988. Linkages between Sexual Activity and Alcohol and Drug Use among American Adolescents. *Family Planning Perspectives* 20(3): 128–136.

Mott, Frank L., and William Marsiglio. 1985. Early Childbearing and Completion of High School. *Family Planning Perspectives* 17(5): 234–237.

Mott, Frank L., and Susan H. Mott. 1984. Prospective Lifestyle Congruence among American Adolescents: Variations in the Association between Fertility Expectations and Ideas Regarding Women's Roles. *Social Forces* 63(1): 184–208.

Namerow, Pearila B., and Judith E. Jones. 1982. Ethnic Variation in Adolescent Use of a Contraceptive Service. *Journal of Adolescent Health Care* 3(3): 165–172.

Namerow, Pearila B., and Susan G. Philliber. 1983. Attitudes towards Sex Education among Black, Hispanic, and Inner-City Residents. *International Quarterly of Public Health* 75(1): 33–38.

Nathanson, Constance A. 1991. *Dangerous Passage: The Social Control of Sexuality in Women's Adolescence*. Philadelphia: Temple University Press.

Newcomer, Susan, and Wendy Baldwin. 1992. Demographics of Adolescent Sexual Behavior, Contraception, and STDs. *Journal of School Health* 62(7): 265–270.

Newman, Lucille F. 1978. The Cultural Perspective. Introduction to *The First Child and Family Formation*, ed. Warren B. Miller and Lucille F. Newman. Chapel Hill: Carolina Population Center, 73–78.

———. 1985. *Women's Medicine*. New Brunswick, N.J.: Rutgers University Press.

Newton, Niles. 1967. Pregnancy, Childbirth, and Outcome: A Review of Patterns of Culture and Future Research Needs. In *Childbearing: Its Social and Psychological Aspects*, ed. Stephen A. Richardson and Alan F. Guttmacher. Baltimore: Williams and Wilkins, 147–228.

Padilla, Amado M., and Traci L. Baird. 1991. Mexican-American Adolescent Sexuality and Sexual Knowledge: An Exploratory Study. *Hispanic Journal of Behavioral Sciences* 13(1): 95–104.

Parker, Barbara, Judith McFarlane, Karen Soeken, Sarah Torres, and Doris Campbell. 1993. Physical and Emotional Abuse in Pregnancy: A Comparison of Adult and Teenage Women. *Nursing Research* 42(3): 173–176.

Paul, Benjamin D., ed. 1955. *Health, Culture, and Community*. New York: Russell Sage Foundation.

Pavich, Emma Guerrero. 1986. A Chicana Perspective on Mexican Culture and Sexuality. *Journal of Social Work and Human Sexuality* 4(3): 47–65.

Pleck, Joseph H., Freya L. Sonenstein, and Leighton C. Ku. 1993. Masculinity Ideology: Its Impact on Adolescent Males' Heterosexual Relationships. *Journal of Social Issues* 49(3): 11–29.

Polit, Denise F. 1989. Effects of a Comprehensive Program for Teenage Parents: Five Years after Project Redirection. *Family Planning Perspectives* 21(4): 164–169, 187.

Polit, Denise F., and Janet R. Kahn. 1985. Project Redirection: Evaluation of a Comprehensive Program for Disadvantaged Teenage Mothers. *Family Planning Perspectives* 17(4): 150–155.

Rapkin, Andrea J., and Pamela I. Erickson. 1990. Acquired Immunodeficiency Syndrome: Ethnic Differences in Knowledge and Risk Factors among Women in an Urban Family Planning Clinic. *AIDS* 4(9): 889–899.

Rindfuss, Ronald R., S. Philip Morgan, and C. Gray Swicegood. 1984. The Transition to Motherhood: The Intersection of Structural and Temporal Dimensions. *American Sociological Review* 49: 359–372.

Romero-Gwynn, Eunice, and Lucia Carias. 1989. Breast-feeding Intentions and Practice among Hispanic Mothers in Southern California. *Pediatrics* 84(4): 626–632.

Rothenberg, P. B., and P. E. Varga. 1981. The Relationship between Age of Mother and Child Health and Development. *American Journal of Public Health* 71: 810–817.

Salazar, Sandra A. 1979. Reproductive Choice for Hispanas. *Health* July/August 1979: 31–36.

Salguero, Carlos. 1984. The Role of Ethnic Factors in Adolescent Pregnancy and Motherhood. In *Adolescent Parenthood*, ed. Max Sugar. New York: Medical and Scientific Books, 75–98.

Scrimshaw, Susan C. M. 1978a. Stages in Women's Lives and Reproductive Decision Making in Latin America. *Medical Anthropology* 2(3): 41–58.

———. 1978b. Family Formation and the First Birth in Ecuador. In *The First Child and Family Formation*, ed. W. B. Miller and L. F. Newman. Chapel Hill: Carolina Population Center, 108–127.

———. 1984. Infanticide in Human Populations: Societal and Individual Concerns. In *Infanticide: Comparative and Evolutionary*, ed. Glenn Hausfater and Sarah B. Hrdy. New York: Aldine, 439–462.

Scrimshaw, Susan C. M., Patricia L. Engle, Lola Arnold, and Karen Haynes. 1987. Factors Affecting Breast-feeding among Women of Mexican Origin or Descent in Los Angeles. *American Journal of Public Health* 77(4): 467–470.

Scrimshaw, Susan C. M., and Elena Hurtado. 1987. *Rapid Assessment Procedures for Nutrition and Primary Health Care: Anthropological Approaches to Improv-*

*ing Program Effectiveness.* Los Angeles: UCLA Latin American Center Publications, University of California.

Shedlin, Michelle G., and Paula E. Hollerbach. 1981. Modern and Traditional Fertility Regulation in a Mexican Community: The Process of Decision Making. *Studies in Family Planning* 12(6/7): 278–296.

Shelley, G. A. 1993. ANTHROPAC Version 4.0. *Practicing Anthropology* 15(3): 30–32.

Singh, Susheela, Aida Torres, and Jacqueline Darroch Forrest. 1985. The Need for Prenatal Care in the United States: Evidence from the 1980 National Natality Survey. *Family Planning Perspectives* 17(3): 118–124.

Smith, Peggy B., Laurilynn McGill, and Raymond B. Wait. 1987. Hispanic Adolescent Conception and Contraception Profiles. *Journal of Adolescent Health Care* 8: 352–355.

Snow, Loudell F. 1993. *Walkin' over Medicine.* Boulder, Col.: Westview Press.

Speraw, Susan. 1982. *Adolescent Motivation for Pregnancy in Three Cultures.* Master's thesis, University of California-Los Angeles School of Nursing.

Spielberg, Steven, director. 1981. *Raiders of the Lost Ark.* Paramount Pictures, Lucasfilm Ltd. Production.

Stack, Carol. 1974. *All Our Kin: Strategies for Survival in a Black Community.* New York: Harper & Row.

Torres, Aida. 1984. Hispanic Adolescents: Focus on Fertility. Paper presented at the 112th annual meeting of the American Public Health Association, Anaheim, Calif., November 15.

Torres, Aida, and Susheela Singh. 1986. Contraceptive Practice among Hispanic Adolescents. *Family Planning Perspectives* 18(4): 193–194.

Upchurch, Dawn M., and James McCarthy. 1990. The Timing of a First Birth and High School Completion. *American Sociological Review* 55: 224–234.

Vega, William A. 1990. Hispanic Families in the 1980s: A Decade of Research. *Journal of Marriage and the Family* 52 (November): 1015–1024.

Ventura, Stephanie J. 1988. Births of Hispanic Parentage, 1985. *Monthly Vital Statistics Report* 36(11): 1–12.

Vinovskis, Maris A. 1981. An Epidemic of Teenage Pregnancy? Some Historical Considerations. *Journal of Family History* 6: 205–230.

Wallace, Helen M., George Ryan, Jr., and Allan C. Oglesby, eds. 1988. *Maternal and Child Health Practices. Third Edition.* Oakland, Calif.: Third Party Publishing.

Weller, Susan C., and A. Kimball Romney. 1988. *Systematic Data Collection.* Qualitative Research Methods Series, vol. 10. Newbury Park, Calif.: SAGE Publications.

Whiting, John W. M., Victoria K. Burbank, and Mitchell S. Ratner. 1986. The Duration of Maidenhood across Cultures. In *School-age Pregnancy and Parenthood: Biosocial Dimensions,* ed. Jane B. Lancaster and Beatrix A. Hamburg. New York: Aldine, De Gruyter, 273–302.

Wiemann, Constance M., and Abbey B. Berenson. 1993. Contraceptive Discontinuation among White, Black, and Hispanic Adolescents. *Adolescent and Pediatric Gynecology* 6: 75–82.

Wilkinson, Doris. 1987. Ethnicity. Chap. 8 in *Handbook of Marriage and the Family,* ed. Marvin B. Sussman and Susan K. Steinmetz. New York: Plenum Press, 183–210.

Williams, Norma. 1990. *The Mexican American Family: Tradition and Change*. Dix Hills, N.Y.: General Hall.

Williams, Ronald L., Nancy J. Bibkin, and Elizabeth J. Clingman. 1986. Pregnancy Outcome among Spanish Surname Women in California. *American Journal of Public Health* 76(4): 387–391.

World Fertility Survey. 1980. Country Reports 17. *The Mexico Fertility Survey, 1976–1977*. March.

Zabin, Laurie S., and Sarah C. Hayward. 1993. *Adolescent Sexual Behavior and Childbearing*. Vol. 26. Developmental Clinical Psychology and Psychiatry Series. Newbury Park, Calif.: SAGE Publications.

Zambrana, Ruth E., Christine Dunkel-Schetter, and Susan C. M. Scrimshaw. 1991. Factors Which Influence Use of Prenatal Care in Low Income Minority Women in Los Angeles County. *Journal of Community Health* 16(5): 283–295.

Zayas, Luis, Steven P. Schinke, and David Casereno. 1987. Hispanic Adolescent Fathers: At Risk and Underresearched. *Children and Youth Services Review* 9: 235–248.

Zelnik, Melvin, and John F. Kantner. 1974. The Resolution of Teenage First Pregnancies. *Family Planning Perspectives* 6(2): 74–80.

———. 1979. Reasons for Non-Use of Contraception by Sexually Active Women Aged 15–19. *Family Planning Perspectives* 11(5): 289–296.

———. 1980. Sexual Activity, Contraceptive Use, and Pregnancy among Metropolitan Area Teenagers: 1971–1979. *Family Planning Perspectives* 12(5): 230–237.

Zelnik, Melvin, John F. Kantner, and Kathleen Ford. 1981. *Sex and Pregnancy in Adolescence*. Beverly Hills, Calif.: Sage Publications.

# Index

Abortion: by Latinos, 31–32, 129, 173n.1; legalization of, 10; norms proscribing, 14; repeat abortions, 2; statistics on, 9; by white adolescents, 31

Acculturation: and gender-role attitudes, 24; and language use, 175n.4; of Latina adolescent mothers, 63–67, 69; and prenatal care, 101–102, 108–109; and sexuality, 32–33. *See also* Norms

Acculturation scale, 175n.4

Adolescent fathers. *See* Fathers

Adolescent fertility. *See* Fertility

Adolescent mothers. *See* Latina adolescent mothers

Adolescent pregnancy: anthropological perspectives on, 18–22; and children of teen mothers, 12–13; and focus on individual, 159–160, 163; historical normalcy of, 20–21; medical interventions for, 18; medical risks of teen childbearing, 11; medicalization of, 5; as minority issue, 13–14, 173n.1; positive aspects of, 156; problem of, in U.S., 9–11, 156, 157, 161–162; public cost of, 13; reasons for, 18; relevancy of middle-class programs for poor teen mothers, 18; repeat pregnancies, 126–128, 130–132, 152–153, 177n.7; as response to bleak life options, 6, 161; social and economic risks of, 11–14; social organization and successful adolescent childbearing, 21–22; and socioeconomic constraints, 160–164; statistics on, 9, 10, 13, 126–127; as test of love and commitment, 144–146; and values, 157–159. *See also* African American adolescent pregnancies; Latina adolescent pregnancies; Prevention of repeat pregnancy; Prevention programs

Adoption, 10, 69, 157, 159

Adult status, and fertility, 19, 22, 34

AFDC, 11, 76–77, 110, 119, 134, 152

African American adolescent pregnancies: link to minority status, 13–14, 173n.1; and low birth weight, 33, 106; positive aspects of, 156; relevancy of middle-class programs for, 18; repeat pregnancies, 126; research on, compared with Latina adolescent pregnancies, 4, 5, 29; social organization supporting, 21; statistics on, 13

African American adolescents: birth rates to, 30; contraceptive use by, 31, 123, 129; economic support from baby's father, 82; sexual behavior of, 30–31; transition events of, 96

African Americans: alternate life-course strategies of women, 17; attitude toward sexuality and marriage, 26; fathers of babies born to teenagers, 82; in Los Angeles, 47–48; median age at transition events

African Americans (*continued*)
for women, 15–16; median years
of education completed by, 16
Age: of Latina adolescent mothers, 68,
69; at menarche, 20, 119
Aguirre-Molina, Marilyn, 173n.1
Aid to Families with Dependent Chil-
dren (AFDC), 11, 76–77, 110, 119,
134, 152
AIDS. *See* HIV/AIDS
Alan Guttmacher Institute, 10
Alicia, 58, 125, 166
Alternate life-course strategies, 17–18
Amaro, Hortensia, 28
Ambivalent mother, 150, 154
Amelia, 135–136
América, 58, 81–82, 147, 165–166
Ana, 73, 147, 152
Anglos. *See* headings beginning with
White
ANTHROPAC, 46, 88
Anthropological perspective on ado-
lescent pregnancy, 18–22, 163–
164
Asians in Los Angeles, 26
Aurora, 66, 75

"Bad woman" versus "good woman"
stereotype, 27–28, 89–90, 96, 98
Bangladesh, 20, 22
Battering. *See* Spouse abuse
Bergen, Candace, 177n.3
Bernstein, Gerald S., 174n.6
Biculturalism and biculturation, 24,
175n.4. *See also* Acculturation
Birth. *See* Childbirth
Birth control. *See* Contraceptive use
Birth outcomes: case studies on, 109–
113; of Latinas, 33, 109–113; and
prenatal care, 105
Birth rates to adolescents, 30, 35
Birth weight: of African American
adolescent births, 33, 106; of Latina
adolescent births, 33, 105–106,
107; and prenatal care, 105–106; of
white adolescent births, 33
Blacks. *See* headings beginning with
African American

Blanca, 56–57, 77, 81–82, 86–87,
124, 125, 133, 144, 146, 147, 165
Breast-feeding plans, 107–109
Burton, Linda M., 96

California: births to Latinas in, 33;
documented versus undocumented
immigrants in, 35–36, 50, 77,
124–125, 174n.4; economic decline
in, 50; education of Latinos in, 25;
illegitimate birth rates to Latina
adolescents in, 30; Latino population in, 175n.3; Proposition 187 in,
36, 174n.4; public cost of adolescent pregnancy, 13. *See also* East
Los Angeles Repeat-Pregnancy
Prevention Project; Los Angeles;
Los Angeles County (LAC)
California Community Foundation,
38–39
Carina, 66
Carmen, 57, 124–125, 133–134, 166
Carolina, 134
Case studies, 66, 73–74, 75–76, 109–
113, 133–136, 144–146, 152–154
Catholic church, 23, 27, 48, 49, 155
Central America, 64–70, 77–80, 84,
88, 106, 108, 115, 121, 175n.6
Child abuse and neglect, 12
Child care, 160, 162, 163
Childbirth: and infant complications,
106–107; and maternal complica-
tions, 107; median age at first
birth, 15, 16; type of delivery, 107.
*See also* Birth outcomes; Birth
rates to adolescents; Birth weight;
Latina adolescent mothers
Children of teen mothers, problems
of, 12–13
*Chola* lifestyle, 1, 2, 73–74, 86–87,
110
Claudia, 66
Clinton, Bill, 9
Condoms, 117, 120, 130–133, 136,
138–142, 176n.2. *See also* Contra-
ceptive use
Contraceptive use: abstinence, 136,
159; by African American adoles-

cents, 31, 123; attitudes toward
contraceptive methods, 137–144;
case studies on, 109–110, 112–
113, 133–136; condoms and foam,
117, 120, 130–133, 136, 138–142,
176n.2; continuation of, over time,
129–130; and contraceptive plans,
116, 117–118, 129; Depo-Provera,
138–142, 153, 177n.5, 177nn.2–3;
factors affecting, 133; failure rates
of contraceptive methods, 132–
133; Hewlet Project on, 174n.7,
177n.1; IUDs, 136–140, 148,
177n.5; and knowledge about
contraception, 115, 117; by Latina
adolescent mothers postpartum,
120–121, 129–148; by Latina adolescents, 31, 123–124; and Latino
cultural values, 23, 27–28; in less-
developed countries, 5; NOR-
PLANT, 53, 138–142, 175n.6,
177nn.2–3; oral contraceptives,
111, 117, 120, 123, 130–137, 138–
142; plans for, 116, 117–118; and
prevention of repeat pregnancies,
18, 115–121; problems in measurement of, 130; reasons for
refused or discontinued contraceptive use, 133, 144–148; in Scandinavian countries, 158; side effects
and medical protocol, 133–137;
social constraints on, 144–148; and
switching of contraceptive methods, 130–133; types of contraceptive methods, 115, 117; by white
adolescents, 31, 123
Cooksey, Elizabeth C., 173n.1
Cost of adolescent pregnancy, 13
Country of birth: and birth weight,
106; of Latina adolescent mothers,
63–67, 69; and prenatal care, 101–
102, 108–109. See also Central
America; Latin America; Mexico
Cristina, 83
Cubans, 31
Culture: and adolescent pregnancy,
18–22, 163–164; fertility and
adult status, 19, 22, 34; as heuristic

device, 173n.4; historical normalcy
of adolescent childbearing, 20–21;
Latino cultural values, 22–29,
155–156, 163–164; social organization and successful adolescent
childbearing, 21–22

Dalkon Shield, 177n.5
Data analysis, 42, 45, 46, 176n.9
Data collection methods: data analysis,
42, 45, 46, 176n.9; data-collection
forms and variables, 167–168;
Hewlett Project, 42–45, 175n.1;
informal interviews, 43, 44;
LARFPC Project, 41–42; medical
record review, 43–44; participant
and direct observation, 44–45;
postpartum ward surveys, 41–42;
quantitative data methods and
variable definition, 169–171;
sources of data, 5–6; surveys, 41–
43, 175n.2; systematic data collection in 1992, 45–46; triangulation
method, 6
Davis, Kingsley, 10
Depo-Provera, 138–142, 153, 177n.5,
177nn.2–3
Documented immigrants, 35–36,
174n.4
Domestic violence. See Spouse abuse
Dropouts. See Education
Drown (Joseph) Foundation, 38–39
Drug users, 113, 125
Duration of maidenhood, 20

Early childbearing. See Adolescent
pregnancy; African American adolescent pregnancies; Latina adolescent mothers; Latina adolescent
pregnancies
East Los Angeles Repeat-Pregnancy
Prevention Project: clients of
family planning clinic, 52; data collection for evaluation of, 5–6, 40–
46; effectiveness of, in prevention
of repeat pregnancy, 114–128; in
family planning clinic, 36–40, 50–
56, 114; funding sources for, 37;

East Los Angeles (*continued*)
Hewlett Project, 39–40, 41, 42–45, 62, 175n.1, 175n.8, 177n.1; high-risk case management, 38–39, 58–59, 86; hospital personnel, 51–52; hospital setting described, 35–36, 50–56; LARFPC Project, 37–38, 41–42; loss to follow-up at one year, 121; loss to follow-up at two years, 121–126; postpartum care, 37–38, 40, 41, 118–119, 121, 176n.5; program retention studies, 121–126, 176n.5; protection of human subjects in, 46; and repeat pregnancies, 126–128; research team, 56–61, 165–166; researcher's personal background and biases, 59–61; staff of family planning clinic, 52, 174n.5; target groups for, 35, 36, 39; and teen outreach workers (TOWs), 37–38, 39, 42–45, 53–58, 114, 117, 125–128; waiting area of family planning clinic, 52–53. *See also* Latina adolescent mothers

Economic risks of adolescent pregnancy, 11–14

Economic support: for African American adolescent mothers, 82; for Latina adolescent mothers, 81–83, 119

Education: access to, 160, 163; childcare facilities at schools, 74; early school leaving by Latinos, 16, 24–26, 70, 71–75, 161; as goal of Latina adolescent mothers, 87–88, 96, 119; lengthy period of, in industrialized countries, 21; median years of education by ethnicity and race, 16; as path out of poverty, 161

El Salvador, 64, 65, 67, 109, 175n.6

Elena, 73

*Eleven Million Teenagers: What Can Be Done About the Epidemic of Adolescent Pregnancies in the United States,* 10

Employment. *See* Occupations

"Entered without inspection" (EWI), 36

Erickson, Pamela I., 59–61, 97, 166

Ethnic self-identification, 63–66

EWI. *See* "Entered without inspection" (EWI)

Extended families, 83–84

Family: and Latino cultural values, 23–24, 155–156, 163–164. *See also* Marriage

Family planning. *See* Contraceptive use; East Los Angeles Repeat-Pregnancy Prevention Project

Fathers: of babies born to teenagers, 12, 34, 77–85, 113, 119; of Latina adolescent mothers, 84, 85

Feminist movement, 22, 24

Fertility: adolescent fertility rate, 10; and adult status, 19, 22, 34; of children of teen mothers, 13

Flores, Bettina, 23, 25, 28–29, 155, 156, 163

Foam. *See* Contraceptive use

Food and Drug Administration, 177n.5

Forrest, Jacqueline D., 15, 92, 94

Future plans, of Latina adolescent mothers, 87–88, 96, 119

Gangs, 1, 2, 73–74, 86–87, 125

Gender roles: and Latinos, 23–24; perceptions of, by Latina adolescent mothers, 88–92

Gloria, 110, 112

"Good woman" versus "bad woman" stereotype, 27–28, 89–90, 96, 98

Guatemala, 65, 66, 67, 75, 109

Guttmacher Institute, 10

Hamburg, Beatrix A., 20

Hayward, Sarah C., 9

Health care: access to, 160; crisis in Los Angeles, 50, 165, 166, 174n.2, 176n.1; medical interventions for adolescent pregnancy, 18. *See also* Postpartum care; Prenatal care

Henshaw, Stanley K., 31

Hewlett Foundation, 39–40, 174n.7
Hewlett Project, 39–45, 61, 174n.7,
    175n.1, 175n.8, 177n.1. *See also*
    Latina adolescent mothers
H-HANES. *See* Hispanic Health and
    Nutrition Examination Study
    (H-HANES)
High-risk case management, 38–39,
    58–59, 86
High-risk mother, 86–87, 150–151,
    154–155
Hispanic Health and Nutrition Exami-
    nation Study (H-HANES), 31
Hispanics. *See* Latinos; and headings
    beginning with Latina
Historical normalcy of adolescent
    childbearing, 20–21
HIV/AIDS, 3, 57, 165, 166, 173n.4,
    175n.7, 176n.8
"Homemaker complex," 88–91
Housewife-mother, 149–150, 153,
    155–156. *See also* Marriage
Hurtado, Aida, 173n.1
Hurtado, Elena, 6

Illegal immigrants. *See* Undocu-
    mented immigrants
Illegitimate birth rates, 10, 30
Immigrants: documented versus
    undocumented, 35–36, 50, 77,
    124–125, 174n.4; in Los Angeles,
    47–48, 166
Immigration and Naturalization Ser-
    vice, 36, 76
Immigration Reform and Control Act
    (IRCA), 36, 50
India, 22
Industrialized countries, 20–21
Informal interviews, 43, 44
Inocencia, 75–76
Institute of Medicine (IOM), 99,
    104–105
Intercourse. *See* Sexual behavior
Interviews, 43, 44. *See also* Data col-
    lection methods
IOM. *See* Institute of Medicine (IOM)
IRCA. *See* Immigration Reform and
    Control Act (IRCA)

Isabel, 76
IUDs, 136–140, 148, 177n.5

Jamieson, Pat, 35
Japan, 20
Jencks, Christopher, 14, 15
Jobs. *See* Occupations
Jorge, 39, 58–59, 77, 166
Joseph Drown Foundation, 38–39

King, Rodney, 50, 174n.1
Kunitz, Stephen J., 5

LAC-USC Women's and Children's
    Hospital. *See* Women's and Chil-
    dren's Hospital
Lancaster, Jane B., 20
Language: and acculturation, 175n.4;
    and birth weight, 106; and breast-
    feeding plans, 108; and contracep-
    tive knowledge and use, 115; of
    Latina adolescent mothers, 63–
    67, 69
LARFPC Project, 37–38, 41–42
Latin America, 16, 19–20, 23, 25, 64,
    65, 67, 69. *See also* Central
    America; Mexico; and specific
    countries
Latina adolescent mothers: accultura-
    tion of, 63–67, 69; age of, 68, 69;
    and birth outcomes, 105, 109–113;
    and birth weight of babies, 105–
    106; breast-feeding plans of, 107–
    109; characteristics of, 63–98; com-
    plications following childbirth, 107;
    contraceptive knowledge and use
    postpartum, 115–119; contracep-
    tive plans of, 116, 117–118, 129;
    contraceptive use postpartum, 120–
    121, 129–148; country of birth of,
    63–67, 69; economic support from
    baby's father, 81–83, 119; education
    of, 70, 71–75, 87–88, 96, 119; ethnic
    self-identification of, 63–66; future
    plans of, 87–88, 96, 119; Hewlett
    teens compared with other Latina
    adolescent mothers, 62–63, 64; and
    infant complications, 106–107;

Latina adolescent mothers (*continued*)
language of, 63–67, 69; list and
brief description of select cases, 1–
3; living arrangements of, 83–84,
85, 119; long-term follow-up of,
177n.1; as low income, 76–77, 125–
126; marriage of, 77–79, 111, 113,
149–150, 153, 155–156; mobility
of, 124; occupation of, 75–76, 119;
parents of, 84–85; pathways to
motherhood, 149–156; perceived
social support for, 84–86; perceptions of women's roles, 88–92;
postpartum care for, 118–119, 121,
176n.5; pregnancy history of, 68,
69; and pregnancy planning, 68, 69,
71, 105, 175–176n.7; prenatal care
for, 99–113; psychosocial problems
of, postpartum, 120; relationship to
baby's father, 77–83, 113; repeat
pregnancies of, 126–128, 152–153,
177n.7; reproductive plans of, 118,
176n.3; and retention studies, 121–
126, 176n.5; risk status at postpartum, 86–87; sexual behavior postpartum, 119–120; social support
for, 83–86; subjects in research
study, 175n.1; summary of research
findings on, 97–98; telephone
service for, 124; and transition
events, 92–97, 98; type of delivery,
107. *See also* Latina adolescent
pregnancies
Latina adolescent pregnancies: abortion used to terminate, 31–32, 129,
173n.1; and acceptance of teenage
motherhood, 28–29; and adoption,
69; characteristics of, 4; compared
with teen pregnancy among African American and white populations, 4, 5, 29; history of, 68, 69; as
planned pregnancies, 68, 69, 71,
105, 175–176n.7; and prenatal
care, 99–113; relevancy of middle-
class programs for, 18; repeat pregnancies, 126–128, 152–53, 177n.7;
research methodology on, 5–6;

statistics on, 13, 30, 35, 126–127.
*See also* Latina adolescent mothers
Latina adolescents: abortion rate of,
31–32, 129, 173n.1; acculturation
of, and sexuality, 32–33; birth outcomes of, 33, 109–113; birth rates
to, 30, 35; contraceptive use by, 31;
early school leaving by, 16, 24–26,
70, 71–75, 161; hardships of, 2–4;
research on reproductive behavior
of, 29–34; sexual behavior of, 30–
33, 98; and sexuality, 26–28
Latinas: abortion of Latina women
versus Latina adolescents, 31, 129;
and acceptance of teenage motherhood, 28–29; attitudes toward
sexuality and marriage, 26–28, 33,
96, 98; birth outcomes of, 33, 109–
113; and contraception, 23, 27–28;
cultural values of, 22–29, 33–34,
155–156, 163–164; early marriage
and school leaving, 24–26, 161;
early school leaving by, 16, 24–26,
70, 71–75; gender-role norms and
the family, 23–24; "good woman"
versus "bad woman," 27–28, 89–
90, 96, 98; primacy of motherhood
and marriage, 22–23; and transition events, 15–16, 21, 92–97; use
of term, 173n.1
Latino fathers, 34, 77–85, 113, 119
Latinos: and acceptance of teenage
motherhood, 28–29; attitudes
toward sexuality and marriage,
26–28, 33, 96; and contraception,
23, 27–28; cultural values of, 22–
29, 33–34, 155–156, 163–164;
early marriage and school leaving,
16, 24–26, 161; family of, 23–24;
father of babies born to teenagers,
34, 77–85, 113, 119; gender-role
norms and the family, 23–24; in
Los Angeles, 47–50; primacy of
motherhood and marriage, 22–23;
sexual behavior of, 30–33; use of
term, 173n.1; variations among
different subgroups of, 29–30

Less-developed countries, 4–5, 20, 22.
*See also* Central America; Latin
America; Mexico; and other specific countries
Leticia, 144–146
Letters for follow-up, 124, 126
Living arrangements: of Latina adolescent mothers, 83–84, 85, 119;
postpartum living arrangements,
119
Lorinda, 57–58, 147, 166
Los Angeles and Los Angeles County:
area of, 47; births in, 35; disparity
of wealth in, 50; economic decline
in, 50; as "global city," 47–48;
health care crisis in, 50, 165, 166,
174n.2, 176n.1; health facilities in,
102–103; Latinos in, 47–50; Mexican Americans moving out of East
Los Angeles, 86–87; population of,
47, 174n.2; violence following Rodney King verdict, 50, 174n.1; Watts
riots in, 50
Los Angeles County–University of
Southern California Women's and
Children's Hospital. *See* Women's
and Children's Hospital
Los Angeles Regional Family Planning
Council, Inc. (LARFPC), 37–38
Los Angeles Women's Foundation, 3
Lover role, 89–92
Low birth weight: among African
American adolescent births, 33,
106; among Latina adolescent
births, 33, 105–106, 107; and pre-
natal care, 105–106, 107; among
white adolescent births, 33
Luker, Kristin, 18, 160, 173n.3, 177n.2
Lupe, 73–74

Machismo, 23–24
Maidenhood, duration of, 20
Mail for follow-up, 124, 126
María, 66, 73
Marianisma, 24
Marin, Gerardo, 175n.4
Marriage: attitudes toward, by ethnic
group, 26; of Latina adolescent
mothers, 77–79, 111, 113, 149–
150, 153, 155–156; Latino cultural
values, 22–23, 26, 28, 155–156; in
less developed countries, 19–20,
22; median age at, 15, 16, 20; in
Mexico, 80–81
Maryland, 82
Medicaid, 11, 13, 76
Medi–Cal, 76, 104, 110, 152
Medical care. *See* Health care; Post-
partum care; Prenatal care
Medical record review, 43–44
Medical risks: of older childbearing,
161; of teen childbearing, 11, 161
Medicalization, 5
Menarche, age at, 20, 119
Menstruation. *See* Menarche
Mexican Americans: abortion by, 31;
attitudes toward sexuality, 27, 28;
birth rate to, 30; and education, 70,
72; and feminist movement, 24;
and gender-role norms and the
family, 24; as largest Latino group,
29; in Los Angeles, 47–50; move
from East Los Angeles, 86–87;
prenatal care for, 102, 110–111;
self-identification as, 64, 66; sexual
behavior of, 30, 32–33; in Teen
Project, 175n.5. *See also* headings
beginning with Latina and Latino
Mexico, 28, 64–73, 75–82, 84, 88, 97,
104, 106, 108, 111, 115
Michigan, 33
Middle-class norms for childbearing,
14–15, 18
Minorities. *See* headings beginning
with African American, Latina, and
Latino
Miscarriages, 2, 9, 153
Mobility of Latina adolescent mothers,
124
Molina, Carlos W., 173n.1
Mothers. *See* Latina adolescent mothers
Mott, Frank L., 126, 128
Multidimensional scaling, 176n.9
*Murphy Brown*, 161, 177n.3

Nathanson, Constance C., 10, 14
National Institute for Child Health
    and Development (NICHD), 165,
    178n.1
Neonatal Intensive Care Unit, 107
Newman, Lucille, 18–19
Nicaragua, 65, 66, 67, 109–110
NICHD. *See* National Institute for
    Child Health and Development
    (NICHD)
Noncompliance, definition of, 2,
    173n.3
Norms: alternate life-course strategies
    among minority populations, 17–
    18; for childbearing, 14–15; his-
    torical normalcy of adolescent
    pregnancy, 20–21; Latino gender-
    role norms and the family, 23–24;
    and pregnancy prevention, 158;
    timing of transition events, 15–17,
    18–19. *See also* Acculturation
NORPLANT, 53, 138–142, 175n.6,
    177nn.2–3

Observation research method, 44–45.
    *See also* Data collection methods
Occupations: of Latina adolescent
    mothers, 75–76, 119; of Latino
    fathers, 83
Oral contraceptives, 111, 117, 120,
    123, 130–137, 138–142. *See also*
    Contraceptive use

Pakistan, 22
Pam. *See* Erickson, Pamela I.
Parental leave, 160
Patricia, 110–111
Perla, 111, 112
Physical abuse, 2, 80, 120
Planned pregnancies of Latina adoles-
    cents, 68, 69, 71, 105, 175–176n.7
Postpartum care, 37–38, 40, 109–110,
    112–113, 118–119, 121, 176n.5
Postpartum ward surveys, 41–42
Poverty, 76–77, 125–126, 155–156,
    160, 163
Pregnancy: median age at, 16. *See also*
    African American adolescent preg-

nancies; Latina adolescent
    pregnancies
Premarital intercourse, 9, 14, 19–20,
    96, 157. *See also* Sexual behavior
Prenatal care: and acculturation, 101–
    102, 108–109; and birth outcomes,
    105, 109–113; and birth weight,
    105–106, 107; and breast-feeding
    plans, 107–109; case studies on,
    109–113; and country of birth,
    101–102, 108–109; definition of
    adequate care, 100; definition of
    inadequate care, 100; importance
    of, 99; inadequacy of, for teens and
    poor women, 99–101; and infant
    complications, 106–107; and
    maternal complications, 107; rea-
    sons for inadequate prenatal care
    among adolescents, 11, 104–105;
    social factors and adequacy of, 105;
    source of, 102–104; and type of
    delivery, 107
Prevention of repeat pregnancy: con-
    traception postpartum, 18, 120–
    121; and contraceptive knowledge
    and use postpartum, 115–119; and
    contraceptive plans, 116, 117–
    118, 129; effectiveness of Teen Proj-
    ect for, 114–128; in family plan-
    ning clinic, 36–40; incidence of
    repeat pregnancy, 126–128, 177n.7;
    limited impact of programs for,
    7–8, 17–18, 159–160; and living
    arrangements postpartum, 119;
    long-term benefits of, 177n.1; and
    pathways to motherhood, 154–
    156; redefinition of criteria for suc-
    cess, 153–154, 177n.1; and repro-
    ductive plans, 118, 176n.3; reten-
    tion studies, 121–126, 176n.5; and
    return for postpartum appoint-
    ment, 118–119, 176n.5; and sexual
    behavior postpartum, 119–120;
    staff response to repeat pregnancies,
    127–128; statistics on repeat preg-
    nancies, 126–128; and switching of
    contraceptive methods, 130–131;
    and values, 157–159. *See also* East

Los Angeles Repeat-Pregnancy Prevention Project; Prevention programs

Prevention programs: different approaches to, 157–159; and focus on individual, 159–160, 163; limited impact of, 7–8, 17–18, 159–160; long-term benefits of, 177n.1; and pathways to motherhood, 154–156; problems of, 156–157; redefinition of criteria for success of, 153–154; and remedies for socioeconomic constraints keeping people in poverty, 160–163; and values, 157–159. *See also* Prevention of repeat pregnancy

*Prometida* (engaged), 72, 80

Proposition 187 in California, 36, 174n.4

Public cost of adolescent pregnancy, 13

Puerto Ricans, abortion by, 31

*Quarentena*, 117

Quayle, Dan, 161, 177n.3

*Quinceañera* celebration, 80–81

Racial discrimination, 160, 163

*Raiders of the Lost Ark*, 3

Rape, 2, 80, 109, 112, 151, 152

Repeat pregnancies, 126–128, 130–132, 152–153, 177n.7. *See also* Prevention of repeat pregnancy

Reproductive transition events, 15–17, 18–19, 92–97

Research methods. *See* Data collection methods

Research team of Teen Project, 56–61, 165–166

Retention in Teen Project, 121–126, 176n.5

Risk status at postpartum, 86–87

*Roe v. Wade*, 10

Rosa, 109, 112–113, 136, 152–153

RU486, 53, 174n.6

SABs. *See* Spontaneous abortions

SAS. *See* Statistical Analysis System (SAS)

Scandinavian countries, 158

Scrimshaw, Susan C. M., 6, 74, 97, 151, 175n.4

Sexual abuse, 2, 12, 80, 120

Sexual behavior: and acculturation, 32–33; by African American adolescents, 30; age at first intercourse, 9, 119; attitudes toward, by ethnic groups, 26, 32; of Latina adolescent mothers postpartum, 119–120; by Latino adolescents, 30–33, 98; Latino attitudes toward, 26–28, 33, 96, 98; median age at, 16; premarital intercourse, 9, 14, 19–20, 96, 157; in Scandinavian countries, 158; statistics on adolescent intercourse, 9; by white adolescents, 30, 32. *See also* Contraceptive use

Sexually transmitted infection (STI), 83, 120, 121, 134, 159. *See also* HIV/AIDS

Side effects of contraception, 133–137

Silverman, J., 31

Sinamon, 75

Social risks of adolescent pregnancy, 11–14

Social support: for Latina adolescent mothers, 83–86; perceived social support for Latina adolescent mothers, 84–86; and successful adolescent childbearing, 21–22

Spielberg, Steven, 3

Spontaneous abortions, 2

Spouse abuse, 2, 80, 120

Statistical Analysis System (SAS), 42, 45, 46

STI. *See* Sexually transmitted infection (STI)

"Student complex," 88–91

Suicide, 12

Surveys, 41–42, 175n.2. *See also* Data collection methods

Sylvia, 109–110, 113, 134–135

Teen outreach workers (TOWs), 37–38, 39, 42–45, 53–58, 114, 117, 125–128

Teen Project. *See* East Los Angeles
    Repeat-Pregnancy Prevention
    Project
Teen Smart Program, 165, 174n.7
Teens. *See* headings beginning with
    Adolescent and Latina adolescent
Telephone calls for follow-up, 124, 126
Timing of transition events, 15–17,
    18–19, 92–97
TOWs. *See* Teen outreach workers
    (TOWs)
Transition events, 15–19, 21, 92–
    97, 98
Triangulation method, 6

Undocumented immigrants, 35–36,
    50, 77, 124–125, 166, 174n.4
University of Southern California
    (USC) Medical and Nursing
    Schools, 35
USC. *See* University of Southern Cali-
    fornia (USC) Medical and Nursing
    Schools

Values and pregnancy prevention,
    156–159
Victim-mother, 151, 155
Vinovskis, Maris A., 10

Watts riots, 50
Welfare programs, 11, 13, 76–77, 110,
    119, 134, 152
White adolescents: abortion rate of, 31;
    birth rates to, 30; contraceptive use
    by, 31, 123, 129; and low birth
    weight infants, 33; median age at
    transition events, 15–16; median
    years of education completed by,
    16; repeat pregnancies of, 126;
    sexual behavior of, 30, 32
Whiting, John W. M., 20
WIC (Women, Infants, and Children)
    program, 76, 110, 152
Wife battering. *See* Spouse abuse
William and Flora Hewlett Founda-
    tion, 39–40, 174n.7
Williams, Norma, 23, 24
Women's and Children's Hospital,
    1, 35–36, 50–56, 165, 173n.1,
    174nn.1–4, 174nn.4–5. *See also*
    East Los Angeles Repeat-Pregnancy
    Prevention Project
Work. *See* Occupations
Worker role, 89–92

Zabin, Laurie S., 9